EXCELLENCE IN PRACTICE Series
Katharine G. Butler, Editor

DYSPHAGIA

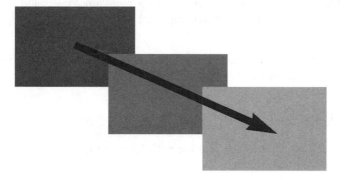

A Continuum of Care

EXCELLENCE IN PRACTICE Series
Katharine G. Butler, Editor

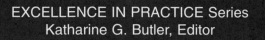

EXCELLENCE IN PRACTICE Series
Katharine G. Butler, Editor

DYSPHAGIA

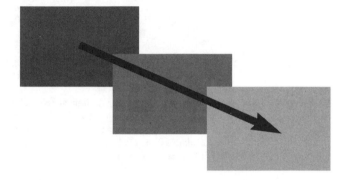

A Continuum of Care

Barbara C. Sonies, PhD
Chief of Speech-Language Pathology
W. G. Magnuson Clinical Center
National Institutes of Health
Bethesda, Maryland

AN ASPEN PUBLICATION®
Aspen Publishers, Inc.
Gaithersburg, Maryland
1997

Library of Congress Cataloging-in-Publication Data

Dysphagia: a continuum of care / [edited by] Barbara C. Sonies.
p.   cm.—(Excellence in practice series)
Includes bibliographical references and index.
ISBN 0-8342-0785-0 (hard cover)
1. Deglutition disorders—Treatment. 2. Deglutition disorders—Patients—Care.
I. Sonies, Barbara C. II. Series.
[DNLM: 1. Deglutition Disorders. WI 250 D9975 1996]
RC815.2.D97 1996
616.85'52—dc20
DNLM/DLC
for Library of Congress
96–42145
CIP

Orders: (800) 638-8437
Customer Service: (800) 234-1660

About Aspen Publishers • For more than 35 years, Aspen has been a leading professional
publisher in a variety of disciplines. Aspen's vast information resources are available in both
print and electronic formats. We are committed to providing the highest quality information
available in the most appropriate format for our customers. Visit Aspen's Internet site for more
information resources, directories, articles, and a searchable version of Aspen's full catalog,
including the most recent publications: http://www.aspenpub.com
Aspen Publishers, Inc. • The hallmark of quality in publishing
Member of the worldwide Wolters Kluwer group

The authors have made every effort to ensure the accuracy of the information herein. However,
appropriate information sources should be consulted, especially for new or unfamiliar procedures.
It is the responsibility of every practitioner to evaluate the appropriateness of a particular opinion in
the context of actual clinical situations and with due considerations to new developments. Authors,
editors, and the publisher cannot be held responsible for any typographical or other errors found in
this book.

Editorial Resources: Brian MacDonald
Library of Congress Catalog Card Number: 96-42145
ISBN: 0-8342-0785-0

Printed in the United States of America

1   2   3   4   5

Table of Contents

Contributors

Evan G. DeRenzo, PhD
Senior Staff Fellow
Bioethics Program
National Institutes of Health
Bethesda, Maryland
Adjunct Lecturer in Bioethics
School of Arts and Sciences
Graduate Program in Biotechnology
The Johns Hopkins University
Baltimore, Maryland
Adjunct Lecturer in Bioethics
Psychology Department
Marymount University
Arlington, Virginia

Madeline Feinberg, PharmD
Clinical Assistant Professor
Director of Elder Health
Department of Pharmacy Practice and
  Science
University of Maryland School of
  Pharmacy
Baltimore, Maryland

Carol M. Frattali, PhD
President
The Garian Group
McLean, Virginia

Gail Gunter-Hunt, BA, MSW
GEM Coordinator and Social Worker
Preceptor, School of Social Work
University of Wisconsin
Madison, Wisconsin

Michelle Johnson, MS, RD, CNSD
Geriatric Specialist, Nutrition and Food
  Services
Wm. S. Middleton Memorial VA
  Hospital
Madison, Wisconsin

Jeri A. Logemann, PhD
Ralph and Jean Sundin Professor
Department of Communication Sciences
  and Disorders
Departments of Neurology and Otolaryn-
  gology—Head and Neck Surgery
Northwestern University
Evanston, Illinois

**Jeri L. Miller, MS, MSc, CCC-
  SLP**
Speech-Language Pathologist
School of Communication Sciences and
  Disorders
McGill University
Montréal, Québec, Canada

Paula C. Ohliger, Esq, OTR
Attorney
California State Bar Association
California Society of Healthcare
   Attorneys
Occupational Therapist
American Occupational Therapy
   Association
San Francisco, California

Adrienne L. Perlman, PhD
Associate Professor
Department of Speech and Hearing
   Sciences
Adjunct Associate Professor
College of Medicine
University of Illinois at Urbana-
   Champaign
Champaign, Illinois

**Beverly Priefer, BSN, MSN, MA,
PhD**
Research Scientist and Geriatric Nurse
   Practitioner
GRECC
Wm. S. Middleton Memorial VA
   Hospital
Madison, Wisconsin

JoAnne Robbins, PhD
Associate Professor and Associate
   Director for Research / GRECC
University of Wisconsin Medical School,
   Department of Medicine
Wm. S. Middleton Memorial VA
   Hospital
Madison, Wisconsin

Margo Schilling, MD
Assistant Professor
GRECC
Wm. S. Middleton Memorial VA
   Hospital
Department of Medicine
University of Wisconsin
Madison, Wisconsin

Justine Joan Sheppard, PhD
Speech-Language Pathologist
Department of Speech and Language
   Pathology and Audiology
Teachers College, Columbia University
New York, New York

Chandar Singaram, MD
Assistant Professor of Medicine
Division of Gastroenterology and
   GRECC
Wm. S. Middleton Memorial VA
   Hospital
University of Wisconsin
Madison, Wisconsin

Kenneth L. Watkin, BA, MA, PhD
Biomedical Engineering
McGill University
Montréal, Québec, Canada

David Watts, MD
Associate Professor
Department of Medicine
University of Wisconsin
Madison, Wisconsin

Forewords

Dysphagia research and practice is one of the most rapidly growing areas of concern in speech-language pathology. Dr. Sonies and her contributing authors are at the cutting edge of research and practice. They bring to this endeavor many years of experience in developing theory and application to the field of swallowing and swallowing disorders.

This text places the diagnoses and treatment of dysphagic patients within the wider context of health care services as they exist today and as they may exist in the future. Readers are provided with current and impending service delivery attributes across the health care continuum, stressing the rapidity with which this continuum is changing in the 1990s and, undoubtedly, into the 21st century. The need for speech-language pathologists and others dealing with dysphagic patients to be able to make critical decisions is central to the multiple themes put forward.

Readers will also find the recurring theme of team approaches to the ethical management of patients with dysphagia. Speech-language pathologists in training (as well as those in allied rehabilitation professions) are faced with devising plans of care which require the input of many providers. Collaboration across settings is of particular importance, as patients move from acute, to subacute, to outpatient or residential rehabilitation programs. As managed care continues to evolve, the cross-disciplinary teams may represent a varying number of professional participants, all of whom must maintain linkages with patients and their families.

The authors provide many case history examples and vignettes which bring to life the problems likely to be encountered in providing services in this very specialized area of care. This text makes apparent the sub-specialties within dysphagia services, focusing on pediatric and adult dysphagia in turn.

In contrast to some other areas of speech-language pathology practice, instrumental procedures for the evaluation and treatment of dysphagia are of singular importance. Carefully described and detailed information is provided regarding the assessment of oral, laryngeal, and pharyngeal swallowing function, including the alternative techniques that can be applied, e.g., videofluoroscopy, flexible fiberoptic endoscopy, ultrasound, electromyography, electroglottography and measurement of the temporal association between respiration and swallowing. For those entering this specialized area of practice, the appropriate use of instrumental procedures requires not only study but supervised practica. Indeed, guidelines and competencies for dysphagia management are currently being finalized by members of the American Speech-Language-Hearing Association.

Widening the scope of the text is an excellent section (Part II) that deals with external issues that influence treatment. Fortunately, the text addresses not only the legal implications in dysphagia practice, providing an important perspective on malpractice issues and relationships with other professionals and payers, but it also addresses clinical ethics. In a seminal chapter, DeRenzo looks at new areas of ethical considerations in the treatment and research of dysphagia, focusing on the secular and sacred nature of certain ethical dilemmas faced by practitioners, persons with dysphagia, and family members. He begins by applying ethical analysis strategies to treatment and research issues in dysphagia, noting that resolving such dilemmas is often not included in clinical or research training. Citing the need for clinicians to uphold the basic biomedical principles of beneficence, respect for persons, and justice, he continues with a consideration of competing moral claims.

DeRenzo brings to the reader's attention the underlying moral values that are embedded within recommendations that professionals consider to be objective and scientific. In a fascinating discussion, he brings together the few major theoretical perspectives, within the philosophical and medical traditions of western medicine. Most readers will not have been exposed to such ethical theories as consequentialism, deontology and virtue ethics, or to feminist and communitarian ethics. He highly recommends that professionals self-monitor their "ethical filters." The reader comes away with a new appreciation of one's professional duties and obligations. The reader also comes away with a three-step blueprint for how to resolve issues through a sensitive approach to the facts, perceptions, and opinions garnered through the fact-finding stage. A review of the societal importance of eating and drinking across cultures brings into focus the importance of social relationships and, frequently, the religious beliefs of those participating in decision making regarding treatment, or withdrawal of treatment, from those with dysphagia. Finally, DeRenzo makes us acutely aware of the exchange of food and drink between individuals, and the consequences of how impairment, interruption, or preclusion of normal eating, swallowing, and communicating affects us all.

Another unusual offering is the chapter on the effects of medications on swallowing, ranging from suboptimal drug therapy that may predispose a patient to oropharyngeal swallowing dysfunction, medications for another medical problem exacerbating concurrent dysphagia, and other direct and indirect causes which may cause or worsen dysphagia. Not only are problems called to the reader's attention, but possible solutions are cited. Medication administration guidelines to reduce risk of esophageal injury are provided, and would be equally helpful to patients and caregivers alike. A complete drug history, including over-the-counter drugs, by a clinical pharmacist is recommended as part of the workup of patients with dysphagia.

The text concludes with some perspectives on the future, and includes professional and education training issues across the spectrum from undergraduate to graduate education, including doctoral and post-doctoral–level possibilities. Logemann contends that the "knowledge base required to be successful as a swallowing therapist is more broad and deep than that necessary in any other area within the speech-language pathologist's domain." While specialists in other areas of speech-language pathology might wish to debate that statement, none would deny the life and death import that is associated with diagnosis and treatment of patients with dysphagia. Not unexpectedly, the claim is made that continuing education is helpful in providing an ever-expanding knowledge base for practicing professionals.

The chapter on instrumental imaging technologies and procedures delves further into many of the new technologies. As Watkin and Miller opine, knowledge of such technologies and procedures requires multidisciplinary knowledge (i.e., radiology, otolaryngology, nuclear medicine, and gastroenterology), and a fusion of effort by the diagnostician and the clinician. Advantages of newly developed procedures as well as their disadvantages provide a fascinating picture of the imagining technologies and future trends. The authors, gazing over the horizon of currently available applications, report on several noteworthy attempts to create three-dimensional imaging systems, attempts in which the authors themselves are intimately involved. The chapter concludes with comments related to the importance of expanding the use of imaging technologies to identify and quantify swallowing disorders, ensuring the accurate assessment and management of patients with swallowing disorders.

On this hopeful note, the editor and authors rest their case. And a powerful case it is. Clinicians and researchers alike will find new information in *Dysphagia: A Continuum of Care*. Editor and author Sonies has chosen well. This text provides a platform from which one can view the continuum of care in its multiple perspectives. The reader will not only understand this rapidly emerging arena of practice more clearly but will also bring to this understanding a level of compassion for the quality of life of patients presenting with dysphagia, be they young or old. The realities, the responsibilities, and the receptiveness to current and future directions in dysphagia diagnosis and treatment is the "critical path" followed by researchers and practitioners alike as they close this volume.

> Katharine G. Butler, PhD
> Research Professor, Communication
>   Sciences & Disorders
> Syracuse University
> Series Editor, *Excellence in Practice*
>   *Series*

Interest in swallowing, swallowing disorders, the diagnosis and management of the dysphagic patient, and research into normal and abnormal swallow and related functions, phonation, and respiration has been growing in leaps and bounds over the last twenty-five years. One of the central professions in this rapidly evolving field is the speech-language pathologist with special expertise in the management of patients with swallowing disorders.

Dr. Barbara Sonies, a world-renowned researcher located at the National Institutes of health, herself a trained speech-language pathologist, has gathered around her experts from many of the disciplines involved in the clinical care of patients with dysphagia. Hence, there are contributors not only from her chosen profession but also from bioethics, elder health, social work, nutrition, the law, nursing, gastroenterology, pediatrics, and biomedical engineering: a diverse group. The scope of the coverage reflects both the sophistication of the technologies that are brought to bear on the clinical diagnosis of a patient but also the wide-reaching consequences of long-term disability. The topics reflect the maturation of thought and philosophy surrounding the whole topic of dysphagic research, diagnosis, and management.

A few years ago, diagnosis and treatment were the key elements of the subject. No mention was made of health care delivery subtleties, ethical or legal issues, or the wider implications to the whole patient of medications that themselves might cause, worsen, or improve the swallowing process or worsen gastrophageal reflux. A discussion of the many technologies available to evaluate the patient with dysphagia (videofluorography, the "gold standard," ultrasound, fiberoptic endoscopy, electromyography, 3D ultrasound) reflects the burgeoning of technologies in general and dysphagia evaluation in particular. Future implications and the need for continuing education are stressed.

Dr. Sonies is to be congratulated on the final product contained within the pages of this book. It is an extremely wide-reaching, thoughtful and thorough approach which should be read with great interest by all involved in the diagnosis and management of patients with dysphagia. Clinical and basic science researchers should find this of interest by providing a holistic picture of investigation in the health care setting of the late 1990s.

Bronwyn Jones, FRACP, FRCR
Professor of Radiology
Director, The Johns Hopkins
  Swallowing Center
Editor-in-chief, *DYSPHAGIA*

Preface

The practice area of dysphagia has burgeoned in the last decade. From an era where dysphagia was of little interest, and even avoided, by most practitioners in speech-language pathology and generally neglected by medical practitioners, it has become one of the most widely referred conditions in many clinical, private practice, and hospital-based programs. A wide range of medical specialties such as gastroenterology, otolaryngology, radiology, physical medicine and rehabilitation, internal medicine, dentistry, pharmacy, and surgery are now interested in using their skills to treat patients with swallowing disorders. The types of patients being referred for evaluation and treatment of dysphagia can range from infants to aged adults. These individuals are often sicker and have more complex problems than patients with communication disorders generally seen by speech pathologists. The practitioner needs to be well trained and highly competent to provide treatment to the wide variety of conditions that can cause dysphagia. Since dysphagia is a complex of symptoms that may accompany many and varied diseases (i.e., systemic, neurologic, genetic, developmental, post surgical, or muscular) the knowledge base needed to provide adequate treatment is greatly expanded. A competent practitioner in dysphagia needs to be in continual contact with the emerging trends and must be current in awareness of new technologies and treatments. In addition to understanding the diseases and conditions that can cause dysphagia, the clinician must be apprised of the effects of treatment, both pharmacological and interventional, that can cause dysphagia. To provide adequate care to patients/clients with swallowing disorders requires an expanded knowledge base, special treatment and observational skills, and awareness of new and emerging diagnostic and instrumental procedures. In addition one must be able to interpret symptoms which may be exacerbated or caused by medications. The risks associated with dysphagia practice make it imperative to be knowledgeable regarding the risks and legal implications of treating a complicated patient. Because many of the decisions involving patients with inability to swallow impact on both quality of life and critical decisions that need to be made at the end of life, it is imperative that persons treating dysphagia understand the ethical decisions facing them.

In the current climate where provision of health care is in flux, critical treatment decisions await both the patient and the professional. The first part of this book contains a chapter that addresses these complex health-care issues and provides a model of the health care continuum with suggested critical pathways for patient care.

This book is designed to provide the reader with areas that are essential in understanding dysphagia from the social, societal, legal, spiritual, and technical milieu as well as to understand treatment and technological advances. It also contains a chapter on the educational and training needs of speech-language pathologists who treat swallowing disorders.

It is my sincere privilege to have been able to edit a book with such a wide complement of nationally recognized contributors whose works are at the cutting edge of this complex field.

Barbara C. Sonies, PhD

Acknowledgments

I want to acknowledge Associated Rehabilitation Services of St. Charles, Missouri for providing us with their clinical pathway for CVA patients and to thank Gina L. Shelly, MA, Corporate Discipline Specialist, Speech-Language Pathology Services with Rehab Choice Inc., Associated Rehabilitation Services for her cooperation and efforts.

PART I

Service Delivery

Critical Decisions Regarding Service Delivery Across the Health Care Continuum

Barbara C. Sonies and Carol M. Frattali

Dysphagia management is a continual process—it does not end after the acute stage of medical care. Rather, it proceeds as the patient progresses through one or more levels of care—from subacute, to long-term, home, and outpatient care. This chapter (1) details current changes in the health care system that have redefined the service delivery continuum, (2) discusses the implications of health care restructuring on dysphagia management and the critical need to break traditional molds of practice, (3) proposes a new model of care, (4) discusses ways to measure patient outcomes within the framework of this new model, and (5) offers suggestions for future directions.

CHANGES IN HEALTH CARE DELIVERY

Although the Clinton administration was unsuccessful in effecting sweeping health care reform in the mid-1990s, the enterprise of health care underwent radical change of its own accord without federal government intervention. A very different picture of health care has unveiled itself in a drastically short period—changes that are causing considerable alterations in how clinical assessment and treatment are initiated, planned, and provided.

Managed care currently is at the helm of health care reform, growing and thriving in an economically burdened system as it touts more cost-effective alternatives to traditional models of care. Managed care is a broad term involving systems that integrate the financing and delivery of appropriate health care services, involving, among other arrangements, the following:

- **Health Maintenance Organizations (HMOs)**, which are health delivery systems that offer enrollees comprehensive health coverage for a prepaid fixed fee. HMOs contract with or directly employ practitioners. Enrollees are required to choose from among these providers for all health care services.

- **Preferred Provider Organizations (PPOs)**, which are health care benefit arrangements designed to supply services at a reasonable cost by providing incentives to their enrollees to use designated health care providers. These providers contract with the PPO at a discount based on expected volume levels.
- **Point of Service Plans (POSs)**, which are health plans in which members do not have to choose how to receive services (e.g., whether from HMO- or non-HMO providers) until they need them (i.e., until the point of service). Coverage is greater, however, if network providers are chosen.

The primary objective of managed care, regardless of arrangement, is to provide comprehensive services at a lower cost. Managed care organizations are buyers. If they can buy the same service from one provider at a lower cost as opposed to another, they will do so. Thus, in many cases, the burden of cost cutting is passed along to providers as they enter into risk contracts and play a competitive game of "more for less." Indeed, those providers who can demonstrate objectively that their services are more cost effective than those of the competition will be victors. In effect, managed care has become an antagonist to traditional clinical practice. It rewards business-oriented providers who can predict their costs, measure their outcomes, and render more cost-effective care than their cohorts. It punishes more service-oriented providers who cannot predict their outcomes, may focus only on measuring clinical processes, and render service with disregard for the bottom line.

The infusion of managed care into the health market is largely redefining service delivery. Managed care's cost-conscious focus has produced a new level of care (that is, subacute care), has accelerated the step-down shifting of patient care to involve lower-cost alternatives along the health care continuum, and has encouraged wide-scale integration of services. As well, managed care, as a result of its fixed or discounted payment arrangements, has caused a fixation on measuring, managing, and predicting clinical outcomes. As financiers, managed care agents simply want to know what they are paying for and whether they can get better value for their dollar.

Managed care payment structures and their implications on service delivery are important to understand if one wishes to become a player in the restructured system. Two common payment options include discounted fee-for-service and capitation.

Discounted fee-for-service is a retrospective payment method in which a provider charges for a specific service at a discounted rate after services are rendered. This payment method is attractive as long as the discounted fee covers the practitioner's costs. If the fee does not cover costs, losses magnify as patient volume increases.

A fee-for-service system creates incentives for inefficiency of care. The more services provided, the more practitioners are rewarded with reimbursement. Thus, this arrangement lost ground in the early 1990s. Currently, many managed care organizations are capping fees or establishing maximum allowable charges.

Capitation is a prospectively determined payment method in which providers are paid a fixed amount per member (usually on a per-month basis), regardless of the services the patient requires. This method carries the greatest risk (but also the greatest potential reward) to practitioners. Under this payment method, practitioners must know in advance what it costs to treat selected patient populations. Therefore, the rewards inherent in capitated payments are directly related to the practitioner's ability to predict costs and to continually strive toward more cost-efficient care. Predicting less than the actual cost can result in substantial losses.

In a capitated system, practitioner incentives change radically when compared to fee-for-service arrangements. In a capitated system, practitioners are rewarded for efficiency. It is projected that by the year 2000, capitation will be the predominant method of payment in managed care.

Industry projections suggest that managed care will continue to experience healthy growth well into the future. Enrollment in HMOs rose 12% and enrollment in PPOs rose 19% from 1992 to 1993. Membership in POSs grew almost 33% in the same time period. One of the largest private insurers, Blue Cross/Blue Shield (BC/BS), currently enrolls about 26 million Americans in managed care networks (about 1 in 10 Americans). BC/BS projects that 80% of its enrollees will be in managed care plans by the year 2000 (American Managed Care and Review Association, 1995; Cornett, Klontz, & White, 1994).

Public payers (such as Medicare and Medicaid) also are moving toward managed care. For example, approximately 7% of Medicare beneficiaries are enrolled in managed care plans (100% growth when compared to enrollment in 1990). This percentage is expected to increase dramatically in the future, especially in view of proposed Medicare reforms (Physician Payment Review Commission, 1995).

As the health care system continues to evolve toward managed care, several trends and projections are reported, such as:

- By the year 2000, all health care will be integrated and capitated.
- Only those practitioners who can demonstrate objectively that their services are effective and cost efficient will stay in business.
- Rehabilitation in acute care, as we know it today, is rapidly shifting to the lower-cost alternative of subacute care.
- Aggressive mergers and consolidation will result in fewer players in health care, but these players will be more influential.

- Managed care is de-emphasizing specialized practice and emphasizing general practice. This movement is empowering the multiskilled health practitioner and support personnel who offer services at a lower cost.

Information from investor reports bolsters claims of aggressive restructuring (e.g., Hicks & Miner, 1993). The following observations are noteworthy:

Inpatient rehabilitation growth slows to a 5%-type pace and is bracing for a more competitive environment. Inpatient rehabilitation providers are vulnerable to lower cost subacute competition (e.g., 40% of inpatient rehabilitation patients who have sustained stroke could be treated in a less intensive subacute setting).

Ultimate winners must be able to document cost effectiveness. While most agree that rehabilitation is cost-effective care, there are disparate opinions on the most cost-effective setting in which to deliver that care. The winners will be those who can document and demonstrate cost effectiveness vs. alternative delivery sites.

If practitioners can think beyond the boundaries of their practice setting, whether acute, subacute, long-term, home care, or outpatient, they soon will realize the importance of **seamless** care (continuous across sites) in a cost-conscious and integrated system. If high-quality, cost-effective care is to be provided across the health care continuum, practitioners engaged in dysphagia management must begin to document the value of care across this continuum.

According to Goldsmith (1994), level of care is not synonymous with the setting in which it is provided (e.g., subacute care can be provided in a hospital or long-term care setting). Nevertheless, certain levels of rehabilitative care historically have been provided in distinct environments. In its broadest sense, service delivery has the binary distinction of inpatient and outpatient care. A range of levels of care (described in Appendix 1–A) and distinct settings can be included in the inpatient/outpatient continuum (Figures 1–1 and 1–2). Increasingly, providers are being held responsible for controlling the utilization of service and managing the cost of care delivered at each level. As well, case managers who operate in integrated systems are creating mechanisms to manage and utilize care across the continuum, often through the use of interdisciplinary care paths.

Health care restructuring has and will continue to occur. Given (1) a new philosophy of quality care (i.e., the best for the least), (2) widespread integration of services across settings, (3) a preoccupation with cost/benefit and subsequent service and reimbursement caps, (4) migration of acute care patients to subacute care, and (5) an interdisciplinary care focus, what are the implications for dysphagia management?

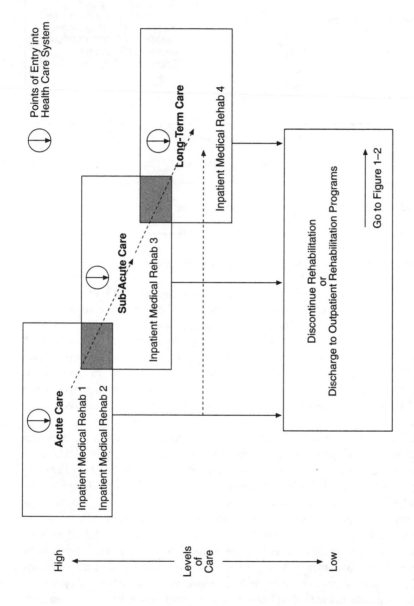
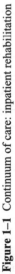

Figure 1–1 Continuum of care: inpatient rehabilitation

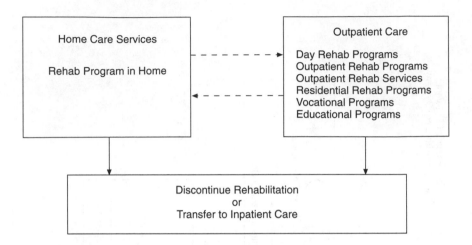

Figure 1–2 Continuum of care: outpatient rehabilitation

IMPLICATIONS FOR DELIVERY OF SERVICE

Because the basic philosophy of health care has changed, practice patterns governing delivery of service will need to accommodate the managed care model. For many, these changes seem radical, but for the few who understand the system, positive strategies can be derived to effectively provide services to persons with dysphagia. Operational restructuring, paired with payment restructuring for services, will force the practitioner to create new cost-effective paradigms of treatment. In fact, practitioners will not survive economically unless they are able to successfully negotiate contracts for services and provide care in the most cost-effective setting.

It will be exceedingly difficult to insist that expensive instrumental procedures be performed on all patients or that multiple videofluorographic swallowing studies be conducted to corroborate observed clinical progress. We will have to develop sets of expected clinical outcomes based on age, diagnosis, length of disease, and severity and complexity of condition to substantiate a videofluorographic study. Costs for more expensive treatments will be scrutinized, particularly in acute care and residential rehabilitation settings, and skilled nursing facilities. Acute care is the most expensive form of health care and it may not be feasible to do a labor-intensive diagnostic or instrumental procedure when the medical condition is unstable. Over the last decade, clinicians have had open invitations to treat patients with dysphagia in the nursing home; however, cost containment may force this to change. Patients in skilled nursing or residential rehabilitation facilities who are cognitively impaired or have dementias may derive minimal benefit from dysphagia treatment. For example, provision of dysphagia treatment for patients with Alzheimer's disease may be questioned, denied, or relegated to aides whose services, albeit unskilled, are less costly. Typically, patients who cannot be fed safely or eat orally are placed on tube feedings. In a cost-conscious environment, however, tube feedings (which are more costly and require special formulas, high-tech care, and special equipment) may be denied.

The speech-language pathologist may be told which patients to treat, how to treat them, and how long they can be treated with little concern for treatment efficacy. Nevertheless, case managers are now asking for proof that the treatment is beneficial. The implications here are that practitioners need to develop more rigorous indicators of treatment effectiveness and efficiency based on cost. These indicators of swallowing improvement will take precedence over conjecture, good intentions, indecision, or speculation. Contrary to current practice expectations, the optimal outcome may not be the attainment of a "normal premorbid swallow," but "reduction of aspiration" or a "nutritionally stable patient."

There are little data on functional outcomes of dysphagia management to support a claim that a greater intensity or a longer period of treatment is better. Unless predictors can be identified that link optimal or minimal sessions needed to achieve specific treatment outcomes in specific conditions, the clinician will be given a set number of dollars in which to provide services for a specified period. Whether the patient needs more help or the family is not fully compliant with the home treatment will not matter.

What clinicians will be expected to provide and what they will be expected to deliver in specified periods during the recovery process will be determined by clinicians who are collecting hard data that demonstrate treatment- and cost-effectiveness. Those who provide service will be expected to develop critical pathways for service delivery (described in the following section) and adhere to the regimens developed. We can posit a scenario when service delivery in the acute care setting is limited to a 5-minute chart review, 15 minutes at the bedside for an oral-motor and clinical swallowing examination, and documentation of recommendations for following the patient into the subacute stages. Trained nurses or dietitians may conduct the initial screening in the acute care setting, rather than speech-language pathologists (whose services may be more costly). Instead of assessment by a member(s) of each separate discipline, a cooperative or interdisciplinary team examination (e.g., by the speech-language pathologist, nurse, physician, and dietitian) might be performed at bedside in the acute care setting. Instrumental assessment such as videofluorography may be deferred until the patient is stable or when discharged to long-term or home care. Use of less costly instrumental procedures such as endoscopy or ultrasound may become more prevalent. Group feeding treatments may be supervised by the speech-language pathologist and conducted by an assistant or an aide. The care given to the dysphagic patient will need to be seamless. Records may be forwarded to appropriate personnel as the patient is referred to the lower cost settings so that services are not duplicated as care proceeds along the continuum (see Figures 1–1 and 1–2). Adherence to critical pathways for evaluation and treatment of persons with dysphagia will be required, especially in the managed care environment.

In summary, the implications for service delivery can be summarized as:

- Fewer and shorter sessions;
- Reduced service in acute care settings;
- Nurses or dietitians screening for dysphagia in the acute care setting;
- Provision of initial services in subacute or long-term care settings;
- More services provided in lower cost settings such as outpatient or home care;
- Restricted use of more costly diagnostic instrumental procedures;
- Team evaluations to determine overall treatment objectives;
- Use of assistants or aides for carry-over and feeding activities;
- Use of critical paths; and
- Use of multiskilled providers who can:
  - screen, assess, and treat patients,
  - counsel staff and families, and
  - follow the patient from acute care through transitional services.

A NEW MODEL OF CARE

Within the context of managed care, a new model of care is emerging. Its primary feature is outcome-oriented and cost-effective care that integrates discipline-specific services across the full continuum of care. To ensure that clinical care has these characteristics, case management has come to the fore.

Case management captures the essence of managed care; its primary goal is cost-effective care. The focus of case management is systematic achievement of outcomes within time and resource limitations. Case managers routinely are employed by managed care organizations to control costs. Their job is to assess the needs of each patient, estimate the cost of care, and coordinate efficient care through care plans and care alternatives. The case manager, an integral member of the interdisciplinary team, wears many hats, including manager of cost and quality, facilitator, liaison, gatekeeper, broker, educator, negotiator, and monitor (Pashkow, 1995).

One of the most valuable case management tools available today is the **critical path** (Larkins Hicks and Frattali, 1995). A critical path is a treatment regime, based on a consensus of clinicians and supported ideally by patient outcomes research, that includes only those vital elements that have been proved to positively affect patient outcomes (Kaine, 1993). Included are clinical management tools that organize, sequence, and time the major interventions of nursing staff, physicians, and other health professionals for a particular case type or condition (Zander, 1994). According to Zander (1994), when length of stay is graphed on an axis against an intervention axis, a basic critical path is born.

Critical paths address three deficiencies in current health care management (Zander, 1994):

1. The inability of existing documentation systems to assist clinicians with integrating the work of each clinical discipline;
2. Limitations of the health care system in setting limits on total work load; and
3. Limitations of current care management tools and professional roles that do not recognize clinical, scientific, and technologic advances.

Thus, critical paths, according to Kimball (1993), are designed to:

1. Strengthen the collaborative nature of patient care through mutually agreed-upon outcomes, time lines, and processes;
2. Direct the contributions of all care providers toward achievement of positive patient outcomes;
3. Provide outcome-oriented patient care within a fiscally responsible time frame;
4. Use the resources that are appropriate, in amount and sequence, to the specific case type; and
5. Ensure that critical areas of patient care are carried out.

Critical paths typically follow the same basic format. The time frame for the path forms the top of each column. It usually is expressed in patient days, although the time frame can be expressed as geographic locations (e.g. hospital, long-term care facility) or phases of care along the continuum (e.g., acute, subacute, outpatient, home care). The functional categories of care are listed in the left margin and can include, for example, assessment, consultations, treatments, medications, diet, patient/family education, and discharge planning. The main body of the grid contains specific actions, tests, assessments, and clinical processes that are expected to be completed within a specified period. Any variance from the critical path is documented in designated areas in the medical record.

Exhibits 1–1 and 1–2 provide examples of a critical path for the sequelae of stroke (Exhibit 1–1) in acute care and the more specific interventions for dysphagia and cognitive/communication disorders (Exhibit 1–2). Developed by Rehab

Exhibit 1–1 Completed Ischemic Cerebral Vascular Accident: Critical Path

CVA	Day 1	Day 2	Day 3
Medical Status	☐ History and Physical Exam	☐ Physical exam	☐ Physical exam
	☐ CT Scan	☐ Continue medications as prescribed	☐ Continue medications as prescribed
	☐ EKG	☐ Manage other acute or chronic medical problems	☐ Manage other acute or chronic medical problems
	☐ CXR	☐ DVT Precautions	☐ CBC
	☐ CBC	☐ Echo	☐ SMA7
	☐ PT/PTT	☐ Holter	☐ D/C I & O
	☐ SMA18	☐ Carotid Studies	☐ D/C Foley
	☐ Sedrate	☐ Monitor O₂	☐ VS q 8 hrs and temp
	☐ Mgt. of other medical problems (acute or chronic)	☐ VS q 6 hrs and temp	☐ x1 x2 x3
	☐ DVT Precautions	☐ x1 x2 x3 x4	☐ Administer prescribed medications
	☐ Determine medications	☐ I & O q 8 hrs	
	☐ Maintain basic airway	☐ x1 x2 x3	
	☐ O₂	☐ IV fluids	
	☐ Assess bowel and bladder function	☐ Administer prescribed medications	
	☐ Foley		
	☐ IV fluids		
	☐ VS q 4 hrs and temp		
	☐ x1 x2 x3 x4 x5 x6		
	☐ I & O q 8 hrs		
	☐ x1 x2 x3		
	☐ Neuro consult		

CVA	Day 1	Day 2	Day 3
Swallowing Nutrition	□ Dietary to assess nutritional needs. □ Recommend appropriate means of nutritional intake.	□ SLP to assess swallowing per bedside evaluation, if indicated. □ SLP and radiologist to perform swallowing instrumental assessment, if indicated, within 24 hours. □ May change initial recommendation based upon swallowing instrumental assessment results.	□ SLP Protocol BID. □ Patient continues to safely tolerate diet consistency.
Mobility	□ Maintain good positioning if patient is transferred for tests, etc.	□ Screen for Physical Therapy □ Physical Therapy Evaluation □ Falls Risk Assessment completed □ Patient up in chair bedside only if trunk stability is present	□ PT Protocol BID □ Patient up in chair BID, only if trunk stability is present
Activities of Daily Living	□ Nursing to encourage patient to do what is realistic and safe. □ OT prepares for evaluation as appropriate.	□ OT initial evaluation as appropriate. □ Follow all precautions. □ Refer to other ancillary services. □ OT to discuss the expectations of rehab. process with patient/family.	□ OT to review OT goals with patient/caregiver. □ OT to follow OT protocol. □ OT to begin upper extremities management/program/activities. □ OT to begin Pre-ADL intervention as appropriate.

continues

Exhibit 1–1 continued

CVA	Day 1	Day 2	Day 3
Activities of Daily Living		☐ OT to work closely with physician, speech, physical therapy, nursing, and other team members (ongoing).	☐ OT to begin basic/simple self-care training in bed or at bedside of grooming and self-feeding if safe and introduce/issue AE as appropriate.
Psycho-Social		☐ Patient and/or family will participate in interview designed to assess psychosocial needs. ☐ Review daily goals with significant other and patient.	☐ Patient/family is aware of self-help/support groups.
Financial Resources	☐ Review patient's financial status and sources of funding.	☐ Patient and/or family is aware of care options related to funding status.	
D/C Planning	☐ Family/significant other states desire to take patient home. ☐ Assess family's ability to assist patient in home environment. ☐ Complete checklist on "home" environment needs for function and safety.	☐ Continue to assess family's ability to assist patient in home environment. ☐ Care team, patient, and family to consider alternative care options. ☐ Prepare patient/family/significant other for transitions to levels of care.	

CVA	Day 1	Day 2	Day 3
D/C Planning	☐ Secure patient/family approval to share medical records with each level of care. ☐ Initiate UR review.	☐ Communicate levels of care. ☐ Stress follow-through. ☐ Plan follow-up contact.	
Postural Support/ Contractures	☐ Assess patient's postural needs in all positions ☐ Restraint assessment ☐ Position patient in bed to support affected UE and provide symmetry to trunk and head and encourage weight bearing through spine	☐ Patient/family/staff education on proper positioning in bed and chair/wheelchair ☐ Position patient in bed to support affected UE and provide symmetry to trunk and head and encourage weight bearing through spine	☐ Patient positioned in bed and/or chair to support affected UE and to provide symmetry to trunk and head while encouraging weightbearing through spine ☐ Continue patient education and training on importance of proper positioning in bed, chair and wheelchair
Cognition Communication		☐ SLP to evaluate cognitive/communicative function. ☐ Initiate speech-language therapy, if indicated.	☐ SLP Protocol BID
Wound Care	☐ Assess skin integrity. ☐ Recommend and implement techniques to reduce risk of skin breakdown.	☐ Continue to assess and adjust positioning to reduce risk of skin breakdown.	☐ Continue to assess and adjust positioning to reduce risk of skin breakdown.

Exhibit 1–2 Completed Ischemic Cerebral Vascular Accident (SLP) Dominant Side: Critical Path for Swallowing

CVA	Day 1	Day 2	Day 3
Medical Status			
Swallowing/ Nutrition	☐ Consider non-oral feedings as a means of primary or sole means of nutritional intake.	☐ Assess swallowing function per bedside evaluation. ☐ SLP and radiologist to perform swallowing instrumental assessment, if indicated, within 24 hours. ☐ SLP explains purpose of study to patient and family. Patient and family demonstrate understanding. ☐ SLP and radiologist discuss results and implications of swallowing instrumental assessment. ☐ Patient/family/staff review instrumental assessment results with SLP and demonstrate understanding of recommendations relative to results. ☐ SLP communicates results and recommendations of swallowing instrumental assessment with team.	☐ Patient continues to safely tolerate altered diet consistency. ☐ Patient follows through with safe swallow strategies with maximal prompting. ☐ SLP provides indirect treatment to improve swallow (i.e., thermal application, oral motor exercises, practice of swallow maneuvers, etc.). ☐ Patient/family/staff receive training regarding safe swallow strategies. ☐ Staff/family demonstrate ability to cue patient regarding safe swallow strategies during mealtime with close monitoring of SLP. Strategies may include postural changes, increased sensory input, and/or modification in volume and speed of food presentation.

CVA	Day 1	Day 2	Day 3
Swallowing/ Nutrition		☐ Initiate dysphagia treatment, if indicated. ☐ SLP provides indirect treatment to improve swallow (i.e., thermal application, oral motor exercises, practice of swallow maneuvers, etc.) ☐ Patient tolerates recommended altered diet consistency. ☐ Patient follows safe swallow strategies with maximal prompting.	

continues

Exhibit 1–2 continued

CVA	Day 4	Day 5	Day 6
Swallowing/ Nutrition	☐ Patient safely tolerates recommended altered diet consistency. ☐ Patient continues to demonstrate safe swallow strategies with maximal prompting. ☐ Staff/family continue to demonstrate ability to correctly cue patient regarding safe swallow strategies with moderate prompting from SLP. ☐ SLP provides indirect treatment of improve swallow (i.e., thermal application, oral motor exercises, practice of safe swallow maneuvers, etc.)	☐ Patient safely tolerates recommended altered diet consistency. ☐ Patient demonstrates safe swallow strategies with moderate prompting. ☐ Staff/family continue to demonstrate ability to correctly cue patient regarding safe swallow strategies with moderate prompting from SLP. ☐ SLP provides indirect treatment to improve swallow (i.e., thermal application, oral motor exercises, practice of safe swallow maneuvers, etc.).	☐ Patient safely tolerates recommended altered diet consistency. ☐ Patient continues to demonstrate safe swallow strategies with moderate prompting. ☐ SLP provides indirect treatment to improve swallow (i.e., thermal application, oral motor exercises, practice of safe swallow maneuvers, etc.).

CVA	Week 2	Weeks 3–4
Swallowing/ Nutrition	☐ Patient continues to demonstrate safe swallow strategies with moderate prompting. ☐ Patient safely tolerates pureed foods with thickened liquids. ☐ SLP provides indirect treatment to improve swallow (i.e., thermal application, oral motor exercises, practice of safe swallow maneuvers, etc.). ☐ Family demonstrates ability to correctly cue patient regarding safe swallowing strategies with minimal cues from the SLP.	☐ Patient safely tolerates mechanical soft or normal diet consistency. ☐ Patient continues to demonstrate safe swallow strategies with moderate cues. ☐ SLP provides indirect treatment to improve swallow (i.e., thermal application, oral motor exercises, practice of safe swallow maneuvers, etc.).

CVA	Weeks 5–6	Weeks 7–8
Medical Status		
Swallowing/ Nutrition	☐ Patient follows safe swallowing strategies with minimal assistance. ☐ Family demonstrates ability to independently provide cues to patient ensuring safety of swallow. ☐ Family/patient can independently determine appropriate food consistencies for patient.	☐ Discontinue dysphagia treatment. ☐ Patient considered to be at a modified independent level, perhaps requiring an adaptive device or safety considerations are present.

Courtesy of Rehab Choice, Inc. © STL Management.

Choice, Inc., of St. Charles, Missouri, these critical paths illustrate both the inter-disciplinary nature and the coordination of care across the continuum from acute, to subacute, to long-term care.

The critical path is organized across time (on the horizontal axis) by functional categories (on the vertical axis). The path is designed to move the patient through the various levels of care, from acute care to long-term care or to the home, in a seamless fashion. Although these time frames are approximations of the length of care, acute care usually encompasses the first four or five days, subacute care can range from several weeks to a month, and long-term care generally lasts from five weeks until discharge. The functional categories include medical status, swallow-ing/nutrition, mobility, activities of daily living (ADL), psychosocial status, finan-cial resources, discharge planning, postural support/contractures, cognition/com-munication, and wound care. These functional categories involve the disciplines of medicine (including radiology), nursing, physical therapy, occupational therapy, speech-language pathology, dietary, social work, and other support ser-vices.

On day 1 of acute care, non-oral feeding is considered as a means of nutritional intake. The dysphagia evaluation occurs on day 2, including both bedside and instrumental diagnostic techniques. The interdisciplinary nature of care is re-flected on day 2 with collaboration of speech-language pathologist, radiologist, and patient/family/staff. Interdisciplinary team communication is an integral ac-tivity throughout the critical path. The activities documented throughout the criti-cal path are outcome-oriented (for example, "Patient safely tolerates recom-mended altered diet consistency." "Patient demonstrates safe swallow strategies with maximal prompting." "Patient follows one-step directions with moderate prompting.").

The critical path continues through the subacute and long-term phases of care with less prompting (from maximal, to moderate, to minimal assistance) until the patient is able to consistently demonstrate safe swallowing strategies on a gradu-ated diet of normal consistency. Once the patient is at a modified independent level regarding swallowing and nutrition (that is, requiring nothing more than adaptive eating devices), treatment is discontinued.

Another model of a critical path used in a rehabilitation setting during stroke recovery was developed by the National Rehabilitation Hospital in Washington, D.C. In this model, several professions including medicine, nursing, occupational therapy, and speech-language pathology have distinct responsibilities regarding swallowing and eating, which are staggered over the time of hospitalization. Ten functional categories are outlined and three of these categories include aspects of feeding or swallowing at different observational or interventional levels. The cat-egory health management medical homeostasis includes medical status, endur-ance, and continuity of care, which are rated by the physician in the first 24 hours of patient admission. Within this category, the RN charts nutrition maintenance from time of admission to discharge. Eating is charted under another category called self-care skills, which the occupational therapist rates at 72 hours after admission and until discharge. The RN completes the initial feeding/swallowing screen and refers patients with specific problems in chewing and swallowing to the speech-language pathologist and the therapeutic feeding team if the problems continue after 72 hours. By the end of the first week, the speech-language pathologist will have completed an evaluation, initiated treatment, and discussed therapy plans with the patient and family members. By the fourth week, a summary is expected in preparation for discharge.

Yet another type of critical path, designed as an outcome scale, was developed by the speech-language pathology department at the William Beaumont Hospital in Royal Oak, Michigan (Merson, Rolnick, & Weiner, 1995) (Exhibit 1–3). The Critical-Clinical Pathway Outcome Scale is part of the Beaumont Outcome Software System (BOSS) and was developed to demonstrate change in patient function in an environment of decreasing length of stay in an acute care setting. Dysphagia has been an area in which measurable, positive changes in outcome can be linked to provision of service over a relatively short period. The BOSS scale consists of a critical path with seven scaled values that can be used with patients whose treatment was attempted but could not be completed because of discharge or inability to notify or secure authorization from family or physicians. The last rating on the scale denotes that the patient is ready for the next phase of dysphagia rehabilitation. Because patients may not have actually received direct services, these scales demonstrate operational outcomes at points along the process of intervention, rather than behavioral outcomes as a result of direct clinical intervention.

In 1993, a study of swallow management in patients on an acute stroke pathway was conducted at a 257-bed, urban, community hospital (Odderson, Keaton, & McKenna, 1995). The study's objective was to assess the effects of swallowing management in 124 stroke patients placed on a clinical pathway, and to evaluate whether swallow function on admission can be used as a predictor of length of stay and outcome disposition. A swallow screen was completed within 1 day of admission and before any oral intake. Outcome measures included presence of dysphagia and Functional Independence Measure (FIM) (State University of New York at Buffalo, 1993) scores on admission, occurrence of aspiration pneumonia, length of stay, outcome disposition, and cost-effectiveness analysis. Thirty-nine percent of all patients failed the initial swallow screen and required altered dietary texture and intervention. No patient developed aspiration pneumonia; 21% recovered intact swallowing by discharge; 19% required gastrostomy tube placement. The length of stay was longer for patients with dysphagia compared to patients without dysphagia. In addition, patients with dysphagia were less likely to be discharged to home than were patients without dysphagia, and twice as likely to be discharged

Exhibit 1–3 Critical-Clinical Pathway Outcome Scale

Inpatient-acute care clinical pathway outcome scale describes the completion of critical services provided (assessment, treatment, consultation, and discharge planning) for the patient's medical care.

Scale Value

---

1   Profound (Incomplete Clinical Pathway)
Patient discharged before completion of speech-language or swallow consultation.

---

2   Severe (Incomplete Clinical Pathway)
Speech-language or swallow evaluation was completed but physician and family have not been yet apprised of the results.

---

3   Significant (Incomplete Clinical Pathway)
Evaluation completed and physician was notified of status. The treatment plan has been implemented but family has not been directly contacted.

---

4   Moderate (Incomplete Clinical Pathway)
The treatment is in progress, the evaluation has been completed, and the physician and family have been notified. Determination of the discharge plan has not been accomplished.

---

5   Mild (Incomplete Clinical Pathway)
The treatment program has been completed, and the family and medical staff have been notified of discharge disposition. The continuing care form for outpatient referrals has not been completed.

---

6   Minimal (Incomplete Clinical Pathway)
The treatment program has been completed, and the family and medical staff have been notified of discharge disposition. The continuing care form for outpatient referrals has not been completed.

---

7   Complete Clinical Pathway
The evaluation and treatment have been completed, and the medical staff has been apprised of patient's communication and swallowing status. The discharge plan has been completed and patient is ready for the next phase of rehabilitation. All medical forms and referrals have been completed.

Courtesy of William Beaumont Hospital, Speech-Language Pathology, 1995, Royal Oak, Michigan.

to a nursing home. This study demonstrated that early swallow screening and dysphagia management in compliance with a clinical pathway in patients with acute stroke reduces the risk of aspiration pneumonia, is cost effective, and ensures quality care with optimal outcome.

Clearly, service delivery is directed toward accountability for outcomes using interdisciplinary treatment protocols such as critical paths. The focus on outcomes, however, presents yet another challenge as practitioners are increasingly held responsible for measuring the results of their interventions across the continuum of care and sharing the data with key decision-makers.

MEASURING OUTCOMES ACROSS THE HEALTH CARE CONTINUUM

Outcomes measurement, as reflected in the previously mentioned critical paths, has a new meaning in a restructured and managed health care system. It is currently perceived to be necessary to measure outcomes to obtain third-party reimbursement and even for professional survival as disciplines with overlapping scopes of practice vie for exclusive rights in the system. Those who can demonstrate objectively that their services make a difference and are cost effective (or more cost effective than those of the competition) will be strategically positioned to negotiate managed care contracts or work within managed care arrangements. Patient care outcomes, although simple to understand, are complex regarding their measurement and management, particularly when regarded across a continuum of care.

The concept of outcomes measurement begins with determining desired patient outcomes. These outcomes can be considered along a sequence of the consequences of a disease, disorder, or injury. The sequence involves the outcomes of impairment, disability, and handicap—outcomes that the World Health Organization (WHO) International Classifications of Impairments, Disabilities, and Handicaps (World Health Organization, 1980) defines as the following:

Impairments: Abnormalities or psychological, physiologic, or anatomic structure or function at the organ level. Examples are paralysis and speech, language, hearing, cognitive, and swallowing disorders.

Disabilities: Restrictions or lack of ability manifested during the performance of daily tasks. Disabilities, then, are defined as the functional consequences of impairments. Examples are difficulties in dressing, toileting, money management, and eating for adequate nutrition.

Handicaps: Social, economic, or environmental disadvantages resulting from impairments or disabilities. Handicaps are defined, in large measure, by societal attitudes about individuals with disabilities. Examples are joblessness, dependency, feelings of low self-worth, and social isolation.

Using the example of dysphagia, the WHO typology can be illustrated. A patient with cerebral vascular disease (disease) who has sustained a stroke (disorder) is found, after diagnostic work-up, to have dysphagia (impairment). The dysphagia, which is characterized by aspiration and choking, results in eating difficulties that interfere with adequate nutrition (disability). The disability leads to dependency on caregivers, use of a nasogastric tube, and feelings of low self-worth because of loss of self-sufficiency (handicap).

Unless one believes that assessment findings at the impairment level can be directly interpolated to reveal parallel findings of subsequent disability or handicap, a one-to-one relationship may not exist. In fact, an inverse relationship may be present. That is, one person with a severe impairment may have a mild disability or handicap, whereas another person with mild impairment may have a more marked disability or handicap. Again, using the example of dysphagia, a disability can be reduced if the patient uses compensatory techniques or adapts a diet regimen of, for example, mechanical soft foods and thickened liquids. In fact, the central purpose of speech-language pathology treatment is to reduce the level of disability, and thus, prevent or reduce handicap. Batavia (1992) believes, "with appropriate rehabilitative interventions, an impairment does not necessarily result in a disability. Similarly, with appropriate social and environmental interventions, a disability does not necessarily result in a handicap" (p. 3).

The consequences of stroke as identified previously can be measured, thus, cataloguing three classes of outcome measures. Measures of impairment include traditional diagnostic measures (e.g., Rehabilitation Institute of Chicago (RIC)—Clinical Evaluation of Dysphagia [Cherney, 1994], Penetration-Aspiration Scale [Rosenbek, Robbins, Roecker, Coyle, & Woods, 1996]) and instrumental procedures (e.g., scintigraphy, ultrasound imaging, and videofluoroscopy) (Table 1–1). As we move along the continuum, disability can be measured using the several available functional assessment instruments that evaluate swallowing. An example of a functional swallowing measure is the dysphagia outcome scale developed by William Beaumont Hospital in 1996, and included in the BOSS (Merson et al., 1995). This measure, which rates level of swallowing deficit from profound (parenteral or tube feeding) to normal range (without need for intervention) on a 7-point ordinal scale, is applicable for use across a continuum of care (i.e., acute care, inpatient, and outpatient rehabilitation) (Exhibit 1–4). Finally, measures of handicap include the so-called quality-of-life or wellness measures that are designed as self-administered questionnaires to elicit the perspectives of patients, who are the best judges of their quality of life. Handicap measures often are designed as combined measures of impairment, disability, and handicap, but always as perceived by the patient. Tables 1–1 to 1–4 detail the characteristics of available measures used to characterize impairment, disability, and handicap.

Exhibit 1–4 Dysphagia Outcome Scale

Acute Care, Inpatient, and Outpatient Rehabilitation		
Scale Value	**Level of Deficit**	**Statement of Deficit**
1	Profound	*NPO alternative feeding*, profound oral and/or pharyngeal transit deficit. Medical and mental status impedes PO feeding. Aspiration present or highly likely. Candidate for parenteral or tube feeding only.
2	Severe	*Trial feeding for therapeutic purposes only. Primary parenteral or tube feedings.* Severe oral and/or pharyngeal dysphagia.
3	Significant	*Supplemental tube feeding may be required.* Moderate to severe oral and/or pharyngeal dysphagia. [Dysphagia I* diet with ultra-thick liquids.]
4	Moderate	*At risk for aspiration* with thin liquids; *however, tube feeding is not required.* [Dysphagia I* or II** diet with thickened liquids.]
5	Mild	*Mild oral and/or pharyngeal dysphagia.* Patient may have single sips of thin liquids. [Dysphagia II** diet or soft diet with thick liquids.]
6	Minimal	*Patient may require swallowing strategies*, slight abnormality in oral and/or pharyngeal phase. [Soft or regular diet with thin liquids.]
7	Normal Range	Normal swallow.

*Dysphagia I = Pureed-consistency diet. **Dysphagia II = Casserole-consistency diet.

Courtesy of William Beaumont Hospital, Speech-Language Pathology, 1995, Royal Oak, Michigan.

Table 1-1 Characteristics of Selected Impairment Measures

Source	Title	Description	Reliability/Validity
Sonies, Parent, Morrish, & Baum, 1988	Swallowing Questionnaire	Checklist of 20 items that measure subjective awareness of swallowing difficulty	Discriminates between normal population and various patient populations
Cherney, 1994	Rehabilitation Institute of Chicago (RIC)—Clinical Evaluation of Dysphagia (CED)	Checklist based on findings from clinical examination and VF study	Clinical impressions
Rosenbek, Robbins, Roecker, Coyle, & Woods, 1996	Penetration-Aspiration Scale	8-point interval scales	Kappa coefficients for intra- and interjudge agreement are high
Cherney, 1994	RIC—Clinical Evaluation of Dysphagia— Pediatrics	Based on developmental feeding scales and clinical observations check lists	Clinical impressions

Measurement of Consumer Satisfaction

An often-neglected area of outcome assessment relates to measurement of consumer satisfaction. Requirements of the Joint Commission on Accreditation of Healthcare Organizations (1996) and other regulatory and accreditation directives, which specify the measurement of patient and family satisfaction with services, have facilitated the movement toward patient-centered care. Donabedian (1988), a prominent authority in quality assessment, states:

> Patient satisfaction may be considered to be one of the desired outcomes of care, even an element in health status itself. . . . It is futile to argue about the validity of patient satisfaction as a measure of quality. What-

Table 1-2 Characteristics of Dysphagia Instrumental Procedures

Instrument	Advantages	Limitations	Uses	Comments
Videofluoroscopy or Modified Barium Swallow (Logemann, 1986)	Dynamic real-time study of all phases of swallow. Easy to interpret.	Radiation exposure. Not mobile. Contrast agent cannot be used repeatedly.	Displays complete physiology and anatomy of swallow. Detects aspiration penetration.	The "gold standard"
Fiberoptic nasoendoscopy of swallow (Langmore, Schatz, & Olsen, 1988)	Portable, less expensive; uses regular food with dyes; biofeedback therapy	Discomfort; topical anesthetic; cannot see oral or esophageal phase	Detects laryngeal penetration; laryngeal, and pharyngeal residue, detects aspiration material	Does not visualize actual swallowing behavior; need training to use endoscope
Scintigraphy (Fleming, Muz, & Hamlet, 1990; Humphries, Mathog, Miller, Rosen, Muz, & Nelson, 1987)	Computerized calculation of bolus aspiration and locus of residue	Not readily available; no physiology or anatomy seen; uses radioactive tracers	Quantify aspiration after or during a swallow study	Highly specialized equipment
Ultrasound imaging (Sonies, Parent, Morrish, & Baum, 1988; Shawker, Sonies, & Stone, 1984)	Dynamic real-time study of oral pharyngeal swallow; biofeedback; no radiation	No bony structures seen. Esophageal and pharyngeal phases not seen.	Visualize oral cavity and hypopharynx; durational measures	Safe, portable—good for infants; soft tissues visualized

Source: Reprinted with permission from Sonies, B.C., "Instrumental procedures for dysphagic diagnosis," *Swallowing Disorders: Seminars in Speech and Language,* Vol. 12, No. 3, p. 185–198, © 1991, Thieme Medical Publishers, Inc.

Table 1-3 Characteristics of Selected Disability Measures

Instrument (reference)	Assessment Domains	Aspects of Swallowing Measurement	Assessment Method	Reliability Validity
Barthel Index (Mahoney & Barthel, 1965)	Feeding, grooming, moving to bed, bathing, toileting, walking, stair climbing, bowel and bladder control	Feeding (if food needs to be cut = help)	10 points given for independent; 5 points given for requiring help	Information on reliability unavailable. Scores and changes in scores correlate with clinical judgment.
Katz Index of ADL (Katz, Ford, Moskowitz, Jackson, & Jaffee, 1963)	Bathing, dressing, toileting, transfer, continence, feeding	Feeding	Dichotomous scale of dependence/ independence	High reliability based on unpublished data; correlates with mobility and house confinement after discharge
Patient Evaluation and Conference System (Harvey & Jellinek, 1979, 1981)	Functions related to rehabilitation medicine, rehabilitation nursing, physical mobility, ADL, communication, medications, nutrition, assistive devices, psychology, neuropsychology social issues, vocational educational activity, therapeutic recreation, pain, pulmonary rehabilitation, pastoral care	Swallowing	7-point ordinal scale from dependent to independent function	Studies are ongoing. Preliminary studies found wide range of interrater reliability from .68 to .80. Content and construct validity are reported.

Instrument	Domains	Subscale	Scale	Reliability/Validity
Level of Rehabilitation Scale III (Parkside Associates, Inc., 1986)	ADL, mobility, communication, cognitive ability	ADL Subscale of feeding	5-point interval scale ranging from unable to perform to performs all aspects of feeding independently	Interrater reliability of item ratings ranges from .53 to .70 at admission and from .64 to .76 at discharge. Face validity based on agreement by experts in the field of rehabilitation is reported.
Rehabilitation Institute of Chicago Functional Assessment Scale '95 (Cichowski, 1995)	Functions related to physical medicine, nursing, physical therapy, occupational therapy, communication disorders, psychology, social work, vocational rehabilitation, therapeutic recreation	Chewing/Swallowing	7-point ordinal scale ranging from normal to severe ability	Interrater reliability ranges from .66 to 1 across item scores, with 75% to 100% agreement on most items. Interrater reliability for communication items ranges from .90 to 1.00 ($p<.0001$); 100% on all, except written and pragmatic (97% agreement) and speech production (93% agreement)
Functional Independence Measure, Version 4.0 (State University of New York at Buffalo, 1993)	Self-care, sphincter control, transfers, locomotion, communication, social cognition	Eating: Includes the use of suitable utensils to bring food to mouth, chewing and swallowing, once the meal is presented in the customary manner on a table or tray. Performs safely.	7-point ordinal scale from complete independence to total assistance	Intraclass correlation coefficients range from .89 to .96 for FIM domain scores. FIM item Kappa range: .53 (memory) to .66 (stair climbing). Interrater reliability ranges from .97 to .98 for FIM domain scores; FIM item Kappa range: .69 (memory) to .84 (bladder

continues

Table 1–3 continued

Instrument (reference)	Assessment Domains	Aspects of Swallowing Measurement	Assessment Method	Reliability Validity
				management). Reported face-, construct-, and criterion-related (predictive and concurrent) validity (for minutes of help).
Minimum Data Set for Nursing Home Resident Assessment and Care Screening (Hawes, Morris, Phillips, Mor, Fries, & Nonemaker, 1995)	Cognitive patterns, communication/hearing patterns, physical functioning and structural problems (including ADLs), continence, psychosocial well-being, mood and behavior patterns, activity pursuit patterns, disease diagnoses, health conditions, oral/nutritional status, oral/dental status, skin condition, medication use	Oral/nutritional status: oral problems (chewing problem, swallowing problem, mouth pain), height and weight, nutritional problems, nutritional approaches	Check all that apply, or record (i.e., height, weight)	Based on published field test results, interrater reliability value for functional indicator of eating was .94.

A Performance Status Scale for Head and Neck Cancer Patients (List, Ritter-Sterr, & Lansky, 1990)	Eating in public, understandability of speech, normalcy of diet	Eating in public, normalcy of diet	Total of three ratings (one on each subscale). In each subscale, items are arranged hierarchically to describe a continuum, with total incapacitation at one end to full, normal functioning at the other end	Interrater reliability between research team members was .88 for normalcy of diet, and .78 for eating in public. Interrater reliability for untrained professionals was .84 for normalcy of diet, and .81 for eating in public. Moderate correlations were found when compared with Karnofsky Performance Status Rating Scale (Karnofsky & Burchenal, 1949)
Dysphagia Outcome Scale of the Beaumont Outcome Software System (Merson, Rolnick, & Weiner, 1995)	Feeding	Feeding	7-point ordinal scale from profound deficit (NPO alternative feeding) to normal range (normal swallow)	Currently unavailable
Functional Oral Feeding Measure (Johnson, 1995)	Oral feeding	Oral feeding	7-point ordinal scale from normal to nonfunctional for all nutritional needs	Currently unavailable

Source: Adapted with permission from Frattali, C., Thompson, C., Holland, A., Wohl, C., Ferketic, M. *Manual for the American Speech-Language-Hearing Association Functional Assessment of Communication Skills for Adults (ASHA FACS),* © 1995, American Speech-Language-Hearing Association.

Table 1–4 Characteristics of Selected Handicap Measures

Instrument (reference)	Assessment Domains	Assessment Method
Medical Outcomes Study Health Status Questionnaire (Ware & Sherbourne, 1992)	Physical, role limitations due to physical and emotional problems, social functioning, general mental health, pain, energy/fatigue, general health perceptions	Self-report on 36 items
Duke-University of North Carolina Health Profile (Parkerson, Gehlbach, & Wagner, 1981)	Symptom status, physical function, emotional function, social function	Self-report on 64 items
Sickness Impact Profile (Bergner, Bobbit, Carter, & Gilson, 1981)	Physical ambulation, mobility, body care Psychosocial: social interaction, communication, alertness, emotional behavioral Other: sleep/rest, eating, work, home management, recreational pastimes	Self-report on 136 items
McMaster Health Index Questionnaire (Chambers, MacDonald, & Tugwell, 1982)	Physical: mobility, self-care, communication global physical function Social: General well-being, work/social role, performance, social support and participation, global self-function Emotional: Self-esteem, personal relationships, critical life events, global life events, global emotional function	Self-report on 59 items

continues

Table 1–4 continued

Instrument (reference)	Assessment Domains	Assessment Method
Nottingham Health Profile (McEwen, 1988)	Six domains of experience: pain, physical mobility, sleep, emotional reactions, energy, social isolation Seven domains of daily life: employment, household work, relationships, personal life, sex, hobbies, vacations	Self-report on 45 items
Quality of Well-being Scale (Fanshel & Bush, 1970)	Functional performance: self-care, mobility, institutional-ization, social activities Symptoms and problems	Self-report on 50 items
Functional Status Questionnaire (Jette, Davies, & Cleary, 1986)	Physical: basic and intermedi-ate ADLs Emotional function: anxiety and depression, quality of social interaction Social performance: occupa-tional function, social activities Other: sexual global disability, global health satisfaction, social contacts	Self-report on 34 items

Source: Adapted with permission from P. Larkins Hicks, and C. Frattali, Subacute outcome measurement and critical paths development and use, in *Handbook of Subacute Health Care*, K. Griffin, ed. © 1995 Aspen Publishers, Inc.

ever its strengths and limitations as an indicator of quality, information about patient satisfaction should be as indispensable to assessments of quality as to the design and management of health care systems (p. 1743).

Weisman and Koch (1989) point out that satisfied patients are more likely to follow their practitioners' recommendations for treatment. In addition, research has shown that patient satisfaction (or dissatisfaction) is an indicator of other patient behaviors, such as choice of practitioners or programs, disenrollment, use of services, complaints, and malpractice suits (Ware, 1987). Often, tools designed to elicit patient feedback often are the only channel through which patients can alert providers to their concerns, needs and preferences, and perceptions of treatment.

Patient satisfaction relates to both the technical aspects (e.g., appropriate and accurate use of clinical procedures) and interpersonal aspects (e.g., explaining procedures in easy-to-understand language, showing empathy, giving sufficient time to answer patient's questions) of care, as well as the amenities of care (e.g., convenient location and parking, clinical environment that is attractive and ensures privacy, when needed). According to Donabedian (1980), "A subjective summing up and balancing of these detailed judgments would represent overall satisfaction" (p. 25).

Many commercially available, as well as "home-grown," consumer satisfaction measures have been developed. One that would be of interest to speech-language pathologists was developed by the American Speech-Language-Hearing Association (1989). This measures allows patients to rate, on a 5-point scale from strongly agree to strongly disagree, various aspects and outcomes of the clinical process, including the timeliness of service, the benefit of treatment, qualifications of staff, characteristics of the clinical environment, and the staff's interpersonal skills.

Finally, satisfaction of other "consumers" should be considered in outcome measurement activities. For example, the satisfaction of referral sources (e.g., physicians, other gatekeepers) or payers (e.g., Medicare, HMOs) are important to ensure that they perceive dysphagia management as beneficial (e.g., treatment that enhances the patient's ability to live independently) as well as cost efficient (e.g., treatment that can result in shorter lengths of hospital stays and prevent readmissions, treatment that prevents the need for a home health aide). A dissatisfied referral source can choose to refer to other providers and a dissatisfied payer can deny payment for "unnecessary services." In essence, these consumers can block access to service, which hinders well-intentioned clinicians who want to provide service in the best interest of the patient.

Cost Measurement

As stated at the outset of this chapter, the driving force behind health care restructuring is cost containment. According to Wolf, Cohen, and Arnst (1994), two factors are critical for a managed care program to achieve a profit:

- Lowering the managed care program's cost per unit of service; and
- Controlling the number of units of treatment rendered.

It stands to reason then, that managed care organizations will seek out providers who have a history of providing cost-efficient care as well as proven ability to track and predict their costs, and who can provide service that is more cost effective than that of their competitors. Certainly, in the area of dysphagia management, intervention can result in cost savings that can be tracked and reported. For example, dysphagia intervention could result in shorter lengths of hospital stay, or could prevent hospital readmission resulting from development of aspiration pneumonia. Dysphagia intervention could also prevent the need for more costly interventions, such as nasogastric (NG) tube feeding or the need for a home health aide.

An index of cost effectiveness that is growing in popularity with payers is length of stay efficiency. This index, commonly yielded from data from the Functional Independence Measure (FIM) (State University of New York at Buffalo, 1993) is derived by dividing the change score from admission to discharge on a functional outcome measure by the length of stay. The higher the number derived, the greater the length of stay efficiency. This is considered by many to be a gross and flawed measure of cost/benefit, particularly when the outcome measure uses an ordinal, rather than interval scale. With ordinal scales, it is not known whether the intervals between points are equal. Therefore, it is questionable whether moving from a 2 to a 3 shows less change than moving from a 3 to a 5 on a 5-point scale of independence.

As more outcomes management systems are being automated and made commercially available to providers, more cost data will be aggregated and reported for predictive and comparative purposes. Thus, more answers will be supplied for questions such as, "What is the cost of rehabilitating a patient who has sustained a stroke?" and "Are your services more cost-efficient than your competitors'?"

CONCLUSION

This chapter has furnished the reader with the current state of health care delivery and the changes that will have definite impact on the provider of dysphagia treatment. Different types of service provision and payment structures were presented to aid the reader with making informed decisions regarding the choices available to him or her as a potential patient, another consumer, or practitioner. A model of the continuum of health care was presented, which suggests that dysphagia treatment should be integrated across health care disciplines and flow in a seamless fashion from acute to outpatient care settings.

The implications of managed care on dysphagia management will cause providers to negotiate service contracts on the basis of cost and treatment efficiency, rather than productivity. Acute care treatment for dysphagia most likely will diminish whereas subacute and outpatient services will increase. Collection of outcome data is encouraged to support efficacy and cost containment information needed for proof of quality care. Although there is no single best measure of outcome of quality of care, future programs will need to incorporate measurable progress into any management plan if they expect to be reimbursed for service.

The author's intent was to give the reader information for successful execution of dysphagia programs that will prevent or reduce the disabilities and/or handicaps caused by the inability to ingest food and ensure enjoyment of the pleasures afforded by society during mealtime.

REFERENCES

American Managed Care and Review Association. (1995). Quality, choice, satisfaction. Washington, DC: Author.

American Speech-Language-Hearing Association. (1989). Consumer satisfaction measure. Rockville, MD: Author.

Batavia, A.I. (1992). Assessing the function of functional assessment: A consumer perspective. *Disability and Rehabilitation, 14*, 156–160.

Bergner, M.B., Bobbitt, R.A., Carter, W.B., & Gilson, B.S. (1981). The SIP: Development and final revision of a health status measure. *Medical Care, 19*, 787–805.

Chambers, L.W., MacDonald, L.A., & Tugwell, P. (1982). The McMaster health index questionnaire as a measure of quality of life for patients with rheumatoid disease. *Journal of Rheumatology, 9*, 780–784.

Cherney, L.R. (Ed.). (1994). Clinical management of dysphagia in adults and children (2nd ed.). Gaithersburg, MD: Aspen Publishers.

Cichowski, K. (1995). Rehabilitation Institute of Chicago functional assessment scale—Revised. Chicago: Rehabilitation Institute of Chicago.

Cornett, B.S., Klontz, H., & White, S.C. (1994). Managed care: An overview. In *Managing managed care: A practical guide for audiologists and speech-language pathologists.* Rockville, MD: ASHA, Ad Hoc Committee on Managed Care.

Donabedian, A. (1980). *The definition of quality and approaches to its assessment.* Ann Arbor, MI: Health Administration Press.

Donabedian, A. (1988). The quality of care: How can it be assessed? *Journal of the American Medical Association, 260*, 1743–1748.

Fanshel, D., & Bush, J.W. (1970). A health status index and its application to health services outcomes. *Operational Research, 18*, 1021–1066.

Fleming, S.M., Muz, J., & Hamlet, S. (1990). Practical scintigraphic applications for the dysphagic patient. *Asha, 32*, 72.

Goldsmith, T. (1994). Levels of care. In *Managing managed care: A practical guide for audiologists and speech-language pathologists.* Rockville, MD: American Speech-Language-Hearing Association.

Harvey, R.F., & Jellinek, H.M. (1979). *Patient evaluation and conference system: PECS.* Wheaton, IL: Marianjoy Rehabilitation Center.

Harvey, R.F., & Jellinek, H.M. (1981). Functional performance assessment: A program approach. *Archives of Physical Medicine and Rehabilitation, 63*, 43–52.

Hawes, C., Morris, J.N., Phillips, C.D., Mor, V., Fries, B.E., & Nonemaker, S. (1995). Reliability estimates for the minimum data set for nursing home resident assessment and care screening (MDS). *Gerontologist, 35* (2), 172–178.

Hicks, W.G., & Miner, K.M. (May 19, 1993). *The post-acute spectrum of care.* Cowen & Co.

Humphries, B., Mathog, R., Miller, P., Rosen, R., Muz, J., & Nelson, R. (1987). Videofluoroscopic and scintigraphic techniques. *Dysphagia, 4,* 4–15.

Jette, A.M., Davies, A.R., & Cleary, P.D. (1986). The functional status questionnaire: Reliability and validity when used in primary care. *Journal of General Internal Medicine, 1,* 143–149.

Johnson, A. (1995). *Functional oral feeding measure.* Detroit, MI: Henry Ford Hospital.

Joint Commission on Accreditation of Healthcare Organizations. (1996). *Accreditation manual for hospitals.* Oakbrook Terrace, IL: Author.

Kaine, R. (1993). Practice protocols by a different name are not quite the same. *Hospital Rehabilitation, 2,* 124.

Karnofsky, D.A., & Burchenal, J.H. (1949). The clinical evaluation of chemotherapeutics in cancer. In C.M. MacLoed (Ed.). *Evaluation of chemotherapeutic agents* (pp. 191–205). New York: Columbia Press.

Katz, S., Ford, A.B., Moskowitz, R.W., Jackson, B.A., & Jaffee, M.W. (1963). Studies of illness in the aged. The Index of ADL: A standardized measure of biological and psychological function. *Journal of the American Medical Association, 188,* 94–101.

Kimball, L. (1993). Collaborative care: A quality improvement and cost reduction tool. *Journal of Health Care, 15,* 6–9.

Langmore, S.E., Schatz, K., & Olsen, N. (1988). Fiberoptic endoscopic examination of swallowing safety: A new procedure. *Dysphagia, 2,* 209–215.

Larkins Hicks, P., & Frattali, C. (1995). Subacute outcome measurement and critical paths development and use. In K. Griffin (Ed.), *Handbook of subacute health care* (pp. 143–160). Gaithersburg, MD: Aspen Publishers.

List, M.A., Ritter-Sterr, C., & Lansky, S.B. (1990). A performance status scale for head and neck cancer patients. *Cancer, 66,* 564–569.

Logemann, J.A. (1986). *Manual for the videofluorographic study of swallowing.* San Diego, CA: College-Hill Press.

McEwen, J. (1988).The Nottingham health profile. In S. Walker, R. Rosser (Eds.), *Quality of life assessment and application.* Lancaster, England: MTP Press.

Mahoney, F.I., & Barthel, D.W. (1965). Functional evaluation: The Barthel index. *Maryland State Medical Journal, 14,* 61–68.

Merson, R.M., Rolnick, M.R., & Weiner, J. (1995). *The Beaumont outcome software system (BOSS).* West Bloomfield, MI: Parrot Software, Inc.

Odderson, I.R., Keaton, J.C., & McKenna, B.S. (1995). Swallow management in patients on an acute stroke pathway: Quality is cost effective. *Archives of Physical Medicine and Rehabilitation, 76,* 1130–1133.

Parkerson, G.R., Gehlbach, S.H., & Wagner, E.H. (1981). The Duke-UNC health profile: An adult health status instrument for primary care. *Medical Care, 19,* 806–828.

Parkside Associates, Inc. (1986). *Level of rehabilitation scale III.* Park Ridge, IL: Author.

Pashkow, P. (1995). Case management of subacute programs. In K. Griffin (Ed.), *Handbook of Subacute Health Care* (pp. 117–127). Gaithersburg, MD: Aspen Publishers.

Physician Payment Review Commission. (1995). *Annual report to Congress.* Washington, DC: Author.

Rosenbek, J.C., Robbins, J., Roecker, E.B., Coyle, J.L., & Woods, J.L. (1996). A penetration-aspiration scale. *Dysphagia, 11,* 93–98.

Shawker, T.H., Sonies, B.C., & Stone, M. (1984). Sonography of speech and swallowing. In R.C. Saunders & M. Hill (Eds.), *Ultrasound annual* (pp. 237–260). New York: Raven Press.

Sonies, B.C. (1991). Instrumental procedures for dysphagia diagnosis. In *Swallowing Disorders: Seminars in Speech and Language, 12* (3), 185–198.

Sonies, B.C. (1994). Dysphagia: A model for differential diagnosis for adults and children. In L. Cherney (Ed.), *Clinical management of dysphagia in adults and children* (pp. 133–152). Gaithersburg, MD: Aspen Publishers.

Sonies, B.C., Parent, L.J., Morrish, K., & Baum, B.J. (1988). Durational aspects of the oral-pharyngeal phase of swallow in normal adults. *Dysphagia, 3*, 1–10.

State University of New York at Buffalo, Research Foundation. (1993). *Guide for use of the uniform data set for medical rehabilitation: Functional independence measure.* Buffalo, NY: Author.

Ware, J. (1987). Measuring the quality of care: The patient satisfaction component. Presented at the National Conference on Quality Assurance in Ambulatory Health Care, Chicago, IL.

Ware, J., & Sherbourne, C. (1992). The MOS 36-item short form health survey. (SF-36). *Medical Care, 30*, 473–483.

Weisman, E., & Koch, N. (1989). Progress notes: Special patient satisfaction issue. *Quality Review Bulletin, 15*, 166–167.

Wolf, K., Cohen, M.S., & Arnst, D.J. (1994). Managed care: Costs and risks. In *Managing managed care: A practical guide for audiologists and speech-language pathologists* (pp.15–20). Rockville, MD: American Speech-Language-Hearing Association.

World Health Organization. (1980). *International classification of impairments, disabilities, and handicaps.* Geneva: World Health Organization.

Zander, K. (1994). Critical pathways. In M.M. Melum & M.K. Finioris (Eds.), *Total quality management: The health care pioneers* (pp. 305–314). Chicago: American Hospital Association.

Appendix 1–A

Descriptions of Levels of Rehabilitative Care

Inpatient programs:

Inpatient medical rehabilitation 1: This level of care is short term and rendered in general acute care hospitals, general medical/surgical wards, trauma centers, and intensive care units. Patients are acutely ill and medically unstable.

Inpatient medical rehabilitation 2: This level of care is provided in rehabilitation units of acute care hospitals and freestanding medical rehabilitation facilities. It is provided to persons who are still medically fragile, have severe functional limitations, require 24-hour medical support, and have the potential to benefit from a coordinated, intensive, interdisciplinary rehabilitation program. Patients typically can tolerate 3 hours of rehabilitation per day.

Inpatient medical rehabilitation 3: This level of care is less intensive, facility-based rehabilitation. Twenty-four–hour rehabilitation nursing care and coordinated, interdisciplinary rehabilitation services are provided within a nursing facility that has a comprehensive inpatient rehabilitation program. This level of care is provided to patients who have potential for significant functional gains, but who are demonstrating improvement at a rate of less than every 2 weeks and require 24-hour institutional support.

Inpatient medical rehabilitation 4: This level of care is provided in many nursing homes. It consists of intermittent and individual, rather than intensive and comprehensive, rehabilitation services, with an emphasis on improvement in

Source: Adapted with permission from the American Rehabilitation Association (formerly National Association of Rehabilitation Facilities), *Medical Rehabilitation: What It Is and What It Is Not,* © 1988.

functional status or prevention of deterioration of function. Patients progress at a very slow rate and require 24-hour nursing care and physician availability.

Outpatient programs:

Rehabilitation programs and services delivered in the home: This level of care is delivered primarily through home health agencies, and secondarily through hospital outpatient departments or outpatient rehabilitation facilities. Patients are medically stable, require only periodic attention from a rehabilitation physician, and continue to have achievable rehabilitation goals.

Day rehabilitation programs: This level of care is appropriate for individuals who can benefit from intensive interdisciplinary rehabilitation services, but who do not require 24-hour medical and nursing services. Often provided in comprehensive outpatient rehabilitation facilities (CORFs) or the outpatient departments of rehabilitation hospitals or acute care hospitals with rehabilitation units, day rehabilitation programs provide an intense level of coordinated therapies by multiple disciplines 4 to 6 hours per day.

Outpatient rehabilitation programs: This level of care is provided to patients who travel from their homes or other residential settings to outpatient centers in CORFs, outpatient departments of rehabilitation or acute care hospitals, or other outpatient rehabilitation facilities. Comprehensive rehabilitation services are provided under a coordinated interdisciplinary plan of treatment. Therapy is generally less than 5 days per week and usually is provided no more than 3 hours per day.

Outpatient rehabilitation services: This level of care typically is provided at the end of an overall treatment program. It is distinguished from outpatient rehabilitation programs because services are provided by individual clinicians as needed, and plans of treatment are developed by each involved professional.

Residential rehabilitation programs: Transitional living centers, community reentry programs, or independent living centers provide this level of care. Residential programs focus on returning the patient to the community and independent living. A plan of treatment is developed by an interdisciplinary rehabilitation team, and coordinated therapies and other rehabilitation services are provided 5 to 6 hours per day. Patient participation typically extends from 6 to 18 months.

Vocational and educational rehabilitation programs: These outpatient programs focus on return to work or school, rather than medical rehabilitation. They usually are included in vocational rehabilitation centers, special education programs, public or private schools, vocational schools, residential programs, developmental centers, hospitals, or outpatient rehabilitation facilities with work/vocational evaluation, work hardening, or educational programs.

CHAPTER 2

A Team Approach to Ethical Management of an Elderly Patient with Dysphagia

JoAnne Robbins, Beverly Priefer, Gail Gunter-Hunt, Michelle Johnson, Chandar Singaram, Margo Schilling, and David Watts

A central goal of dysphagia team intervention is to restore or maximize swallow function. This goal, which team members and patients mutually accept and which is so fundamental, may not always be explicitly defined. The rationale for restoring or maximizing swallow function may likewise seem obvious: The ability to swallow is an important determinant of patient quality of life. This relationship has been studied relatively little because it is so basic. Yet, a recent study of cancer patients found a strong correlation between dysphagia grade and quality of life (Loizou, Rampton, Atkinson, & Brown, 1992).

The relationship between swallow function and quality of life is complex. Eating involves not only the intake of nourishment, but sensory, social, psychological, and cultural experiences. In a recent analysis of these broader dimensions of non-oral eating, the loss of normal eating ability was associated with depression, altered body image, and disruption of normal cues regarding appetite and satiety (Padilla & Grant, 1985).

A few studies have examined the effects of dysphagia treatments on quality of life. These have involved techniques such as photoablation (Barr & Krasner, 1991) or surgical management of malignant dysphagia (Teichgraber, Bowman, & Geopfert, 1986). Improvements in dysphagia are associated with improved quality of life. Although evaluation of the impact of dysphagia team interventions on the quality of patients' lives awaits further study, promoting patient quality of life is clearly a central goal of the interdisciplinary dysphagia team. Interventions, whether dietary or sociocultural, should be tailored to patient preferences. This is particularly important in the care of elderly patients, for whom impaired swallowing might be only one of several functional losses they are experiencing.

The case report presented largely reflects the efforts of members of a specialized geriatric swallowing/nutrition clinic. With the mission of serving a geriatric population, the team members are aware of the need to continually assess dysphagia and its related problems in the context of the patient's current medical diagnosis and functional limitations. The team follows the basic principles of geriatric assessment: (1) use observational skills, (2) avoid causing distress or indignity, (3) evaluate physical, mental, and social function, (4) uncover signs of disease, and (5) eliminate iatrogenic factors (Williams, 1994). Understanding the difference between illness and disease is essential to the treatment of elderly people, with function rather than disease as the focus. When a diagnosis does need to be made, it usually can be made more effectively regarding the elderly patient by reversing the usual order of the diagnostic thought process: from searching for etiology first to considering the functional impact first. The following case serves to illustrate these principles. An interdisciplinary dysphagia team evaluation and plan of management of a chronically ill patient with multiple diseases and impaired quality of life are presented.

CASE STUDY

In 1989, Mr. P presented to his local hospital with a 2-month history of dysphagia, mouth fullness, and weight loss. He was diagnosed with squamous cell cancer of the tongue. His past medical history was remarkable for pneumonia, hip fracture, and cervical spondylosis. He had a long history of alcohol and tobacco use. Mr. P underwent right hemiglossectomy and radical neck dissection for T3N1M0 squamous cell cancer of the tongue in September 1989. A swallow study, conducted postoperatively, revealed inability to hold a bolus in the oral cavity until told to swallow, severe delay in onset of the pharyngeal swallow response, reduced swallow response when it did occur, no epiglottal movement, decreased hyoid and laryngeal elevation, and severe aspiration. An esophagram showed no reflux. A percutaneous endoscopic gastrostomy (PEG) was placed and the patient was discharged to a nursing home and put on a diet of tube feedings of two cans Sustacal four times daily and NPO status. His course between 1990 and 1992 was complicated by gastrostomy tube (g-tube) malfunctions, noncompliance with tube feedings, alcohol consumption while on pass from the nursing home (three–four beers/day), two episodes of aspiration pneumonia, and repeated requests to resume a more independent lifestyle including resumption of oral intake.

In 1992, a videofluoroscopic swallow study was performed on an outpatient basis at the request of the otolaryngology department. The study findings indicated safe swallowing on only two consistencies: thick liquids and pureed. Thus, it was recommended that Mr. P consume thick liquids and pureed foods orally and receive the remainder of his nutrition through the g-tube. Four weeks later, he returned for outpatient reevaluation because of weight loss. He stated he was not ingesting thick liquids because of their lack of appeal. The nursing home was advised to increase hydration through the tube, and an appointment to our outpatient, geriatric swallow/nutrition clinic was scheduled specifically to consider expansion of Mr. P's oral intake.

GERIATRIC, RESEARCH, EDUCATION, AND CLINICAL CENTER (GRECC)* SWALLOW/NUTRITION CLINIC: STRUCTURE AND FUNCTION

An interdisciplinary team of gerontologists conduct a weekly outpatient clinic to evaluate and treat dysphagia in older individuals. The core team members, a speech pathologist, nutritionist, and geriatric nurse practitioner, evaluate new patients during their initial clinic visit. Members of the extended team, including a gastroenterologist, social worker, pharmacist, and neurologist, evaluate the patient during a follow-up clinic visit as deemed necessary by team members. Mr. P's experience as a patient in our clinic will be presented by each discipline; that is, history related to each relevant team member's area of expertise and the interaction of the patient with each team member are described, including the team plan, its execution, and outcome(s). The chapter concludes with a geriatrician discussing relevant clinical issues.

Social Service

Mr. P, a 76-year-old divorced World War II veteran, is a retired construction worker and farmer with a 10th grade education. He has six adult children, four sons and two daughters, with whom he has very little contact. He lives in a proprietary nursing home in Illinois, where his only visitors are his sister and her children. The sister, who visits frequently, is designated his next of kin. Her husband is a resident of the same nursing home where Mr. P lives. Mr. P has little contact with his two other siblings.

Mr. P smokes one package of cigarettes daily and reports his current alcohol intake to be an occasional beer. His sister, who accompanied him to his GRECC swallow/nutrition clinic visit, stated that he had chronically abused alcohol for all of his adult life. According to the sister, Mr. P's alcohol intake contributed to his alienation from his family and decreased only after his surgery and subsequent nursing home admission.

Mr. P reported a great deal of dissatisfaction with his nursing home environment. He wanted to live in his own home and manage his own care. He only occa-

---

*GRECCs are "centers of excellence" designed for the advancement and integration of research, education, and clinical achievements in geriatrics and gerontology into the healthcare system of the Veteran's Administration.

sionally participated in activities in the nursing home, choosing instead to sit and smoke cigarettes and watch television. Mr. P was dissatisfied with his diet, especially pureed foods. He also did not like the feeding tube and requested to have it removed. He reported that he felt depressed and thought nothing could help change this situation. Mr. P had rejected the idea of relocation to a different nursing home or group home, stating to family and the swallowing team that he would be interested only in relocating home. A modified Carroll rating scale was administered and Mr. P scored 15/25, which is indicative of depressed mood. The modified Carroll rating scale (Greenberg & Drinka, 1990) is a depression screening instrument adapted from the longer Carroll rating scale (Carroll, Feinberg, Smouse, Rawson, & Greden, 1981). A score greater than 5 (out of 25) suggests possible depression and the need for a more comprehensive evaluation of the person's mood.

Mr. P's sister indicated that she believed the nursing home was the best option for her brother despite his dissatisfaction. She reported that he had not adequately cared for himself when he lived alone and said that his needs were being met at the nursing home. The impressions of the social worker at the GRECC swallow/nutrition clinic were as follows:

1. Mr. P has limited social support due to estrangement from his children and his sister's preoccupation with her own husband's illness. Mr. P had not developed an informal support system with any residents in the nursing home.
2. Mr. P was dissatisfied with his living arrangement, yet he was unable to live independently and unwilling to consider relocation to a different facility.
3. Mr. P's mood needed further evaluation to rule out depression.

Nutrition

On his first visit to our clinic, Mr. P stated that his diet at the nursing home consisted of pureed foods with thickened liquids and included 480 cc of a tube feeding product. The tube feeding product was isotonic and contained fiber. Although unsure of the amount, Mr. P felt the water he was receiving through his feeding tube was insufficient. The results of laboratory tests did not reflect dehydration. He complained of pain at the site of his PEG, and also complained of nausea and diarrhea from the tube feedings, which were administered via gravity drip. These complaints were continuous throughout his relationship with the GRECC swallow/nutrition team and negatively influenced his willingness to receive feedings through his PEG.

The nutritional assessment completed during his second visit to our clinic showed that with the exception of his weight being 80% of what was considered "ideal" for his height (Miller, 1985), all other nutritional parameters (Table 2–1) were within normal limits. His current weight, 117 lbs, reflected a 6-lb loss in 2 months. He continued to receive a pureed diet with thickened liquids. However, because of complaints of nausea, his tube feedings were decreased to 240 cc a day. A 3-day diet record completed by the nursing home staff showed Mr. P's daily intake to be between 1,100 and 1,250 calories with 45 to 53 g of protein. Based on the Harris-Benedict equation (Harris & Benedict, 1919) this was estimated to meet 75% of his needs.

When Mr. P returned 2 months later, his weight had decreased by an additional 6 lbs (he now weighed 111 lbs) and his serum albumin had dropped to 3.8 mg/dl. He expressed great unhappiness living in the nursing home. In an attempt to increase his oral intake, the nursing home provided Mr. P with foods he reportedly enjoyed and worked toward liberalizing the consistency of the foods. He no longer was receiving thickened liquids and his foods were ground rather than pureed. Despite these modifications, he continued to refuse to eat. The nursing home staff attempted to increase the volume of his tube feedings to compensate for his poor oral intake, yet he refused all but 240 cc a day. It was apparent that his unhappiness with his living situation and the presence of the feeding tube contributed to his refusal to eat.

Speech Pathology/Swallowing

During his first interaction with the swallowing clinician on his first visit to the GRECC swallow/nutrition clinic, Mr. P reported that he had been ingesting ground foods by mouth for the previous 5-week period and also admitted to "sneaking" water by mouth. He expressed total displeasure with his g-tube and great desire to eat as he wished. In fact, he confided that on occasion he would leave the nursing home and walk to a nearby restaurant where he would eat a hamburger.

Table 2–1 Findings of Nutritional Assessment Completed During Second Visit

weight = 117 lb
total lymphocyte count = 1,950
albumin = 3.8 mg/dl
hemoglobin = 13.0 gm/dl
hematocrit = 38.5%

A brief oropharyngeal sensorimotor examination revealed an edentulous oral cavity. Lip seal and mandibular motion were judged adequate for functional swallowing. Range of lingual motion was limited. Voice was rough and reduced in intensity. Maximum phonation time was reduced. Nonetheless, speech production was 95% intelligible.

Videofluoroscopic swallow study was conducted. The patient was challenged with 3 and 5 cc boluses of thin liquid and semi-solid consistency. Aspiration of a small amount (estimated 5% of one liquid) occurred and "deep" penetration of the laryngeal vestibule (not below the vocal folds) was noted on two liquid swallows (Figure 2–1). No semi-solid material was aspirated; however, repeat swallows of the semi-solid were necessary to clear significant amounts of residue from the base of tongue and in the valleculae after the initial swallow (Figure 2–2). Upper esophageal sphincter opening was judged to be restricted with minimal bolus flow through it, and osteophytes were noted at C4–C6.

During the swallow study, in an effort to increase airway protection, the patient was instructed to perform the supraglottic swallow, which comprises the following five steps:

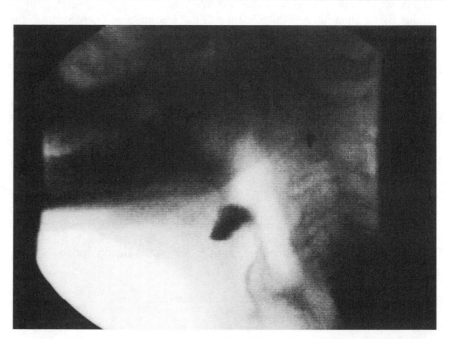

Figure 2–1 "Deep" penetration of liquid with no closure of the laryngeal vestibule—image obtained during first visit to GRECC swallow/nutrition clinic.

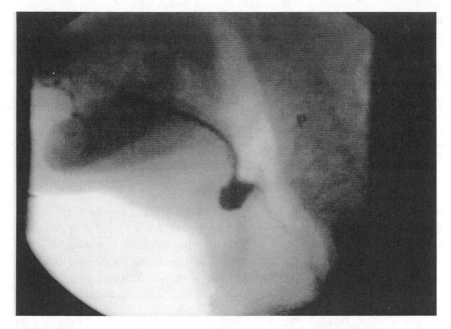

Figure 2–2 Semi-solid residue on tongue and in valleculae after swallowing.

1. Hold breath at level of glottis,
2. Put food in mouth,
3. Swallow,
4. Cough (to clear any material on cords), and
5. Swallow again.

Also, a chin tuck was recommended to provide additional airway protection and to facilitate tongue dorsum to posterior wall contact (Logemann, 1986). Finally, the patient was instructed to hard swallow in an effort to increase intrabolus pressure by more rigorous lingual propulsion.

In light of the aspiration and prior history of recurrent pneumonia, a chest radiograph was obtained upon completion of the swallow study. The radiograph revealed no significant aspiration or pneumonia.

At the conclusion of the initial session, the patient was requested to practice the supraglottic swallow, hard swallow, and chin tuck and was instructed to use these maneuvers during PO intake. Given the results of the chest films, diet recommendations included to continue eating ground and soft foods, and to add moisture in the form of sauces and gravies to facilitate the formation of cohesive boluses and to perhaps increase flow through the oropharynx. Water was permitted in small amounts. An 8-week, follow-up clinic appointment was scheduled.

Upon his return to the clinic, Mr. P complained that his g-tube site was tender and hurt when he ate. Therefore, he ate small amounts to minimize discomfort. Videofluoroscopic reevaluation of swallowing revealed similar findings to those obtained 8 weeks earlier. A small amount of a 3 cc liquid bolus was aspirated (Figure 2–3). A second 3 cc liquid bolus was swallowed without difficulty. Semisolid material required four to five repeat swallows for 3 cc to pass through the upper esophageal sphincter opening, otherwise pooling at the valleculae. Mr. P stated that he only occasionally practiced the maneuvers he was taught during the prior session and did not intend to use them in a rigorous fashion. The risks involved in eating and drinking without practicing the protective maneuvers were explained to Mr. P, including increased risk of choking and pneumonia. Nonetheless, at this visit his lungs were clear. Recommendations included (1) two tube feedings per day, (2) continued PO intake of thick liquids and moist semi-solids, and (3) consultation with a gastroenterologist to examine tube and determine source of continuous discomfort, especially during tube feeding.

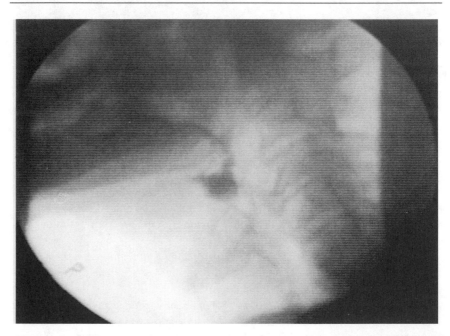

Figure 2–3 "Deep" penetration of liquid in the presence of arytenoid to aryepiglottic fold contact—image obtained during second visit to clinic with patient attempting supraglottic and effortful swallow maneuvers.

When Mr. P returned to the clinic 2 months later for a follow-up visit, he had lost 6 more lbs. He stated he did not want to increase tube feeding. In fact, he wanted more oral intake options because he was receiving mostly pureed foods at the nursing home, despite our recommendations to progress him to semi-solids. No swallow study was performed because there was no basis on which to expect change. Again, Mr. P reported he only occasionally used the supraglottic swallow and chin tuck even though he indicated that he understood the risks, including choking and pneumonia, of not using the maneuvers as previously explained by the swallowing clinician.

Gastroenterology

A Bard-R, 18 Fr. gastrostomy tube was placed using endoscopy (PEG) in 1989, before radical neck dissection for squamous cell carcinoma of the neck. The g-tube was placed at the body of the stomach, pointing toward the pylorus. On re-evaluation 6 weeks after g-tube placement, the position of the tube, patency, and wound healing appeared to be normal, but the patient complained of discomfort on slight movements, even with deep inspiration.

During his visits to the GRECC swallow/nutrition clinic, Mr. P continued to complain of pain at the g-tube site which had continuous, mild to moderate, yellowish discharge. No irritation around the tube site was noted. The team gastroenterologist began Mr. P on a course of metronidazole, 500 mg three times per day and ciprofloxin 500 mg twice per day for 4 weeks with reduction in the amount of discharge. Nonetheless, the patient continued to have similar discomfort at the g-tube site. Mr. P was assessed to have unexplainably more abdominal pain symptoms. The g-tube site and positioning were felt to be within normal limits.

Finally, Mr. P underwent endoscopy for continued complaints of epigastric pain and to rule out recurrent peptic ulcer disease. Endoscopy revealed no peptic ulcer disease, old duodenal healed ulcers, and the g-tube in normal position with no other complications.

Team Staffing

By the end of Mr. P's third clinic visit, team members acknowledged that Mr. P was sending two consistent messages to the team: he wanted his g-tube removed and he wanted to eat only by mouth. The team, however, was uncertain whether Mr. P understood the risks and benefits of that decision. Team members discussed Mr. P's ability to make medical decisions for himself. Mr. P had completed a Durable Power of Attorney for Health Care document before admission to the nursing home. This is a legal document that goes into effect only when the person no longer possesses capacity to make his or her own decisions. The means of determining decision-making capacity is specified according to state law and may vary somewhat from state to state. In Wisconsin, the law dictates that decision-making capacity shall be determined by two physicians or a combination of a physician and a psychologist. At the time he completed this document, Mr. P clearly possessed decision-making capacity. In the power of attorney document, he had named his sister as his "health care agent," the person authorized to make health care decisions on his behalf should he become incapacitated and no longer able to express his wishes. Given Mr. P's mood and his lack of cooperation with his tube feedings, the team requested the GRECC geropsychiatrist to evaluate Mr. P to determine his current capacity to make decisions. The geropsychiatrist's impressions were as follows:

1. Mr. P's thoughts were logical and goal-directed with no evidence of a thought disorder.
2. He was alert and oriented to person (name, not age), place (setting, not the city or state), and time (season, not year, month, or date).
3. His affect was normal with his mood being "pretty good" (per Mr. P) on the day of the evaluation. There was no suicidal ideation.
4. Mr. P was not thought to be clinically depressed. His decreased appetite appeared to be related to discomfort from the PEG rather than depression. Mr. P was taking an antidepressant medication for sleep and the psychiatrist did not see any need to change this.
5. Mr. P was thought to be cognitively impaired because of a Mini Mental State Examination score of 19/30. This questionnaire administered by an interviewer examines the following measures: orientation, registration, attention and calculation, recall, and language. A score below 24 (out of 30) is considered abnormal (Folstein, Folstein, & McHugh, 1975).
6. Despite his cognitive impairment, Mr. P was thought to be competent and to possess decision-making capacity regarding the possible removal of the feeding tube. He understood the risks of aspiration, weight loss, and even death. Clearly, this decision should remain with him and the power of attorney for health care should not be invoked.

Plan of Care and Related Issues

Plan

After the geropsychiatrist declared Mr. P to be competent, the GRECC swallow/nutrition team discussed treatment options with Mr. P. Given Mr. P's wishes to eat orally despite the risks, the team decided to support his decision by establishing the following treatment plan: (1) temporarily withholding his tube feedings for 4 weeks, (2) PO intake ad lib for 4 weeks with the patient understanding that his goal is to maintain his current weight, (3) obtain his weight at the end of 4 weeks, and (4) tube removal if weight remains stable or increases at the end of 4 weeks.

Communication of Plan

Although Mr. P was competent to make his own decisions regarding his health care, he was not totally responsible for his day-to-day care because he lived in a skilled nursing facility. Thus, with respect to Mr. P's swallowing and nutrition needs, he was actually receiving care from two health care teams: the GRECC swallow/nutrition clinic as well as the nursing home team of providers that potentially consisted of a nurse, nursing assistant, physician, social worker, speech and occupational therapists, and nutritionist. Communication was necessary for both health care teams to cooperate with each other and carry out the treatment plan in a consistent manner. Therefore, the GRECC swallow/nutrition team geriatric nurse practitioner, who also serves as the team coordinator, communicated and elicited support from the nursing home staff for our recommended plan. The team speech pathologist/swallowing clinician communicated and elicited support from the nursing-home physician.

Although literature exists on interdisciplinary health care teams (Tsukuda, 1990; Qualls & Csirr, 1988; Drinka, 1991), little information is available on collaborative relationships between two or more such teams. Yet, involvement of multiple health care teams in patient care is becoming more common. As illustrated in Mr. P's case, a resident in a nursing home receives care from a team of providers at his residence and also may receive care at one or more interdisciplinary clinics located in a facility away from the nursing home. Individuals living at home also might receive care at an interdisciplinary clinic such as a geriatrics clinic while simultaneously receiving care from a home health agency team. As in Mr. P's case, one of the teams tends to be more involved on a daily or weekly basis than the other team and may perceive itself as the primary health care team. The GRECC swallow/nutrition team spent a relatively small, infrequent amount of time with Mr. P whereas the nursing home staff spent 24 hours a day over a several-year period with him. In this situation, it is important that information be promptly and accurately transferred between the two teams.

Mr. P had appeared angry about his tube feedings to the swallowing team members. He told the team that the nursing home staff did not dilute his tube feedings or administer them daily as ordered. Upon communicating with the nursing home, the swallow/nutrition team learned that the tube feedings were, indeed, diluted and were given daily, but that the tube was repeatedly found to be disconnected and running into Mr. P's bed. Communication with the nursing home staff helped the team to better understand the patient's weight loss, confirmed his dissatisfaction with the nursing home, and emphasized the need to develop and implement a plan of nutritional care with which Mr. P would comply.

Execution of Plan

When the geriatric nurse practitioner explained the team's rationale for the proposed plan to the nurse in charge of Mr. P's care at the nursing home, she agreed that the plan would be supported and methods to do so were established. The swallow team requested that the patient be weighed daily or every other day. The nursing home could not comply because of staffing constraints. Although their standard of practice was to weigh patients once a month, they did agree to weigh Mr. P weekly during the 4-week period during which he would not receive supplemental tube feedings. Thus, the nursing home agreed to give Mr. P a trial of total oral intake and to remove the feeding tube if he maintained his weight during the 4-week period.

Outcome

The plan was implemented. The patient complied. One month later, Mr. P had lost an additional 2 lbs on oral feedings. Despite the weight loss, he continued to resist the tube feedings and the tube was removed approximately 3 months later. Six months after the tube was removed, Mr. P's weight was 111 lbs, that is, back up to the weight he was on his third swallow/nutrition clinic visit.

CONCLUSION

The swallowing team members became knowledgeable regarding the patient's medical situation, as well as his swallowing, nutritional, and psychosocial status. Treatment approaches were evaluated and adjusted according to the patient's motivation, changing needs, and circumstances. Ultimately, the swallowing interventions were monitored for their physiologic effects (improved nutrition, decreased aspiration) in the context of the patient's quality of life.

Competent patients have a right to refuse treatment, including medically supplied nutrition and hydration, and interventions to improve swallowing function (Pearlman, 1993). Information about treatment options should be presented to patients in a way that conveys respect for their individual desires and preferences. Team members also should be prepared to accept that patients may not desire a "cure," defined as physiologic response to treatment alone.

Tube feeding has come to be viewed as a medical therapy that can be withheld or withdrawn if its burdens outweigh its benefits (Lo & Dornbrand, 1989; Sullivan, 1993). Informed patients, or surrogates for incompetent patients, can decide to forgo tube feeding, although informed consent is often problematic (Krynski, Tymchuk, & Ouslander, 1994; Ouslander, Tymchuk, & Krynski, 1993).

Quill found that restraints were often used to keep incompetent patients from pulling out tube feedings (Quill, 1989). He also noted that many patients who were fed via tubes died in the hospital, particularly those treated for "comfort" only. Assessments of gastrostomy tube feedings, conversely, found good results documented by long-term safety records (Hull, Rawlings, Murray, Field, McIntyre, Mahide, Hawkey, & Allison, 1993), and little negative impact on quality of life was reported (Weaver, Odell, & Nelson, 1993). Clearly, a decision to use tube feedings should be based on patient preferences and careful assessment of likely benefits, not only in physiologic terms, but regarding the patient's quality of life.

REFERENCES

Barr, H., & Krasner, N. (1991). Prospective quality of life analysis after palliative photoablation for the treatment of malignant dysphagia. *Cancer, 68,* 1660–1664.

Carroll, B.J., Feinberg, M., Smouse, P., Rawson, S.G., & Greden, J.F. (1981). The Carroll rating scale for depression. *British Journal of Psychiatry, 138,* 194–200.

Drinka, T.J.K. (1991). Development and maintenance of an interdisciplinary health care team: A case study. *Gerontology and Geriatrics Education, 6* (3), 43–53.

Folstein, M., Folstein, S.E., McHugh, P.R. (1975). Mini-mental state: A practical method for grading the cognitive state of patients for the clinician. *Journal of Psychiatric Research, 12,* 189–198.

Greenberg, J., & Drinka, T. (1990). The modified Carroll rating scale. Unpublished data.

Harris, J.A., & Benedict, F.C. (1919). *Biometric studies of basal metabolism in man.* Washington, DC: Carnegie Institute.

Hull, M.A., Rawlings, J., Murray, F.E., Field, J., McIntyre, A.S., Mahide, Y.R., Hawkey, C.J., & Allison, S.P. (1993). Audit of outcome of long-term enteral nutrition by percutaneous endoscopic gastrostomy. *Lancet, 341,* 869–872.

Krynski, M.D., Tymchuk, A.J., & Ouslander, J.G. (1994). How informed can consent be? New light on comprehension among elderly people making decisions about enteral feeding. *Gerontologist, 34* (1), 36–43.

Lo, B., & Dornbrand, L. (1989). Understanding the benefits and burdens of tube feedings. *Archives of Internal Medicine, 149,* 1925–1926.

Logemann, J.A. (1986). *Manual for the videofluorographic study of swallowing.* (2nd ed.). Austin, TX: Pro-Ed, Inc.

Loizou, L.A., Rampton, D., Atkinson, M., Brown, S.G. (1992). A prospective assessment of quality of life after endoscopic intubation and laser therapy for malignant dysphagia. *Cancer, 70,* 386–391.

Miller, M.A. (1985). A calculated method for determination of ideal body weight. *Nutritional Support Services, 5* (3), 31–33.

Ouslander, J.G., Tymchuk, A.J., & Krynski, M.D. (1993). Decisions about enteral tube feeding among the elderly. *Journal of the American Geriatrics Society, 41,* 70–77.

Padilla, G.V., & Grant, M.M. (1985). Psychosocial aspects of artificial feeding. *Cancer, 55,* 301–304.

Pearlman, R.A. (1993). Forgoing medical nutrition and hydration: An area for fine-tuning clinical skills. *Journal of General Internal Medicine, 8,* 225–227.

Qualls, S.H., & Csirr, R. (1988). Geriatric health teams: Classifying models of professional and team functioning. *The Gerontologist 28,* 372–376.

Quill, T.E. (1989). Utilization of nasogastric feeding tubes in a group of chronically ill, elderly patients in a community hospital. *Archives of Internal Medicine, 149*, 1937–1941.

Sullivan, R.J. (1993). Accepting death without artificial nutrition or hydration. *Journal of General Internal Medicine, 8*, 229–224.

Teichgraber, J., Bowman, J., & Geopfert, H. (1986). Functional analysis of treatment of oral cavity cancer. *Archives of Otolaryngology—Head and Neck Surgery, 112*, 959–965.

Tsukuda, R.A. (1990). Interdisciplinary collaboration: Teamwork in geriatrics. In C.K. Cassel, D.E. Riesenberg, L.B. Sorenson, J.R. Walsh (Eds.), *Geriatric medicine* (pp. 668–675). New York: Springer-Verlag.

Weaver, J.P., Odell, P., & Nelson, C. (1993). Evaluation of the benefits of gastric tube feeding in an elderly population. *Archives of Family Medicine, 2*, 953–956.

Williams, M.E. (1994). Clinical management of the elderly patient. In W.R. Hazzard, E.L. Bierman, J.P. Blass, W.H. Ettinger, Jr., J.B. Halter, Editor Emeritus—R. Andres (Eds.), *Principles of geriatric medicine and gerontology* (pp. 195–201). New York: McGraw-Hill, Inc.

CHAPTER 3

Pediatric Dysphagia and Related Medical, Behavioral, and Developmental Issues

Justine Joan Sheppard

ONTOGENY

It is clear that pediatric dysphagia issues are not simply adult issues on a smaller scale. The interaction of dysphagia with maturation of musculoskeletal, neurologic, and psychologic systems results in complex amalgams of symptoms. Furthermore, the infant's social milieu is unique in its structure and in the complexity of its somatic effects (Als, 1986; Fleisher, 1994; Singer, 1990). In children, as in adults, the characteristics of food-seeking behaviors are determined by the interaction of autonomic cues and environmental inputs. Developmental skills emerge from this interaction during periods of neurologic plasticity that occur for oral and pharyngeal bolus management during the first year of life. Ingestion skills are habituated and paired with self-feeding at the end of the first and into the second years. When the minimum physiologic and environmental requirements for acquisition of ingestion behaviors are not available, therapeutic interventions are needed to provide for nutritional needs, avoid respiratory complications, and facilitate acquisition of skills needed for ingestion.

In infants, emergence of the abilities to ingest nutrients and oral secretions is associated with primitive oral reflexes that provide movement templates for effective reception, formation, and delivery of the bolus into the pharynx (Ingram, 1962; Sheppard & Mysak, 1984). Infants have a plastic neurologic system that facilitates effective and rapid, reward-driven modifications of these patterns. Maintenance of hydration, satiation of hunger, and the associated satisfactions of eating and being fed are potent reinforcers. Modifications occur in response to the specific changes in environmental demands and to the ongoing changes in oral, pharyngeal, and thoracic musculoskeletal relationships (Bosma, 1988; Sonies & Kahane, (1992a, 1992b). In the normal child, the system functions optimally for acquisition of new behaviors associated with swallow during the first year of life (Illingworth & Lister, 1964). The child achieves the basic milestones of mature ingestion behaviors during that period (Newman, Cleveland, Blickman, Hillman, & Jaramillo, 1991; Sheppard & Mysak, 1984). The skills seen during the first year continue to improve and are well established by 2 to 3 years of age (Gisel, 1991; Stolovitz & Gisel, 1991).

PATHOLOGY

The exquisite responsiveness of this system makes the child at once resilient to anatomic, neurologic, and environmental perturbations that are within the child's capabilities for compensation and, when the perturbations exceed those limits, vulnerable to degradation of feeding and swallowing through development of maladaptive movement patterns (Rosenthal, Sheppard, & Lotze, 1995) and feeding phobias (DiScipio, Kaslon, & Ruben, 1978). When these problems are associated with developmental disability, they may persist into adulthood. Pediatric dysphagia, therefore, degrades the process of acquisition of ingestion behaviors as well as their immediate performance, and unresolved issues may become life-long problems. Management of pediatric dysphagia is a formidable task. The clinician must promote the acquisition of behaviors, which, in the normal child, would have emerged naturally from the interaction between physiologic precursors and changing environmental demands. However, in pediatric dysphagia, the precursors are abnormal or have not yet emerged, and the environmental demands may be inappropriate for task acquisition under these atypical circumstances.

Effects of Medical Disorder on Feeding Behaviors

The young child is particularly vulnerable to somatic effects from medical and environmental stressors (Fleisher, 1994; Singer, 1990). Gagging, vomiting, and rumination may become conditioned responses to food, especially when the child has suffered from an illness that involved gastrointestinal distress (Mascarenhas & Dadhania, 1995). Pulmonary and cardiac disorders, when they co-occur with dysphagia, may further degrade swallow or complicate the transition to more normal feeding behaviors. Bazyk (1990) found the duration of the transition from tube to oral feeding in children without specific dysphagia or with resolved dysphagia to range from 2 to 58 days, and to be related to the number of medical complications the child had experienced. The more episodes of cardiac, pulmonary, and gastrointestinal (GI) complications, the longer it took to make the transition. Those children with ongoing dysphagia had longer transitions of 6 to 36 months. Differential diagnosis and management of this complex interaction of physiologic and psychological issues (Hyman, 1994; Rudolph, 1994; Singer, Nofer, Benson-Szekely, & Brooks, 1991) are further complicated by the limited or absent ability of the child to explain his or her symptoms and to respond to instruction.

Developmental Manifestations of Dysphagia Disability

Approaches to pediatric dysphagia differ, depending on the age at which it first becomes apparent and its causes.

Infants and Young Children

Neonates, both premature and full-term, experience difficulties with suckling, swallowing, and the interactions among suckling, swallowing, and breathing. Early interventions may result in the infant achieving normal swallowing abilities, good nutrition, and normally advancing developmental eating skills. Or, these problems may persist in the toddler and young child, causing difficulties with nutrition, airway protection, and ease of eating. Alternately, onset of dysphagia may occur later in infancy as changing musculoskeletal anatomy and environmental demands stress the infant. When the problems persist beyond approximately 6 months, intervention usually is required to resolve difficulties with spoon feeding, cup drinking, chewing, self-feeding skills, and suckling. Thus, the problems of the infant and young child may be transient and may be resolved as feeding behaviors mature. Or, they may be the beginning of chronic disorder.

Older Children and Adolescents

The older child and adolescent with chronic dysphagia present with residuals of early problems plus the added stresses of achieving adequate nutrition for approaching physical maturity. Intervention is needed to aid in developing compensations that will meet their needs as adults, and in modifying maladaptive compensations that may have been habituated at younger ages.

Developmentally Disabled Adults

The adult with developmental disability presents with an amalgam of pediatric and aging issues. Unresolved (i.e., chronic) pediatric problems are complicated by their interaction with the physiologic changes of aging and by the onset of adult disorders. These may include nutritional, gastrointestinal, respiratory, and oral structural problems that are predisposed by the chronic dysphagia or by genetic factors. Although these adults are not technically included in the domain of pediatrics, pediatric perspectives are valuable for understanding and managing their dysphagia (Rubin & Crocker, 1989).

Causes and Consequences of Feeding Disorders

Pediatric feeding disorders fit into two, broad, overlapping categories: (1) those that affect oral, pharyngeal, and esophageal swallowing coordinations (i.e., dysphagia); and (2) those that affect appetite, food-seeking, and behavioral aspects of ingestion (Rudolph, 1994). Attention must be paid to both sets of issues so far as they contribute significantly to the individual's disorder for satisfactory outcomes for nutrition, control of oral secretions, airway protection, ease of eating, and eating skills to be achieved. The first set includes anatomic abnormalities of the nose, mouth, pharynx, larynx, trachea, and esophagus; disorders affecting the coordination of swallowing and breathing; disorders of the neuromotor coordinations of swallowing, including involvement of reflexes, praxis, and neuromuscular competencies; disorders of esophageal peristalsis; infectious and inflammatory disorders of the mucosa; and disorders affecting salivation. The second set includes disorders that exacerbate dysphagia and interfere with its satisfactory resolution. These include primary disorders related to parent-child interactions that may be associated with family stresses that are specific to the child's illness (Handleman, 1995; Singer, 1990; Singer et al., 1991); pediatric psychopathologies (Dowling, 1980; Stroh, Robinson, & Stroh, 1986); sensory deficits; aversions related to lack of appropriate feeding experiences during the critical or sensitive periods of infancy (Illingworth & Lister, 1964); traumatically conditioned dysphagia (feeding phobias), which may be associated with GI disorder, odynophagia, and aspiration (DiScipio et al., 1978); the fatigue and malaise associated with chronic illness (Sheppard & Pressman, 1988); and metabolic and central nervous system diseases (Rudolph, 1994). The consequences of dysphagia and these related medical, behavioral, and developmental issues are (1) failure to thrive; (2) the downward spiral of deglutive and reflux aspiration, frequent respiratory illnesses, and pulmonary disease; (3) increased risk for choking; (4) mealtimes marred by the discomfits of coughing, regurgitation, and food refusal; (5) stressors in the parent-child relationship; (6) failure to advance eating skills; and (7) drooling. Tables 3–1 and 3–2 summarize the causes and consequences of pediatric dysphagia.

EVALUATION

As in the adult model for dysphagia, pediatric evaluation may include both clinical and instrumental components.

Clinical Examination

Assessment of the pediatric patient must be family-centered, multidisciplinary, and team-oriented (Rosenthal et al., 1995). The family members relate the history

Table 3–1 Causes of Pediatric Feeding and Swallowing Disorder

Anatomic Abnormalities
  Skeletal anomalies
  Muscle anomalies
  Infectious and inflammatory disorders of bone and mucosa
Neurologic Pathology
  Oral and pharyngeal reflexes
  Neuromuscular competencies
  Praxic competencies
  Salivation
Behavioral Abnormalities
  Feeding phobias
  Lack of appropriate and timely feeding experiences
  Pediatric psychopathologies
  Atypical parent-child interactions
  Sensory deficits

and symptoms and, using description, inference, and demonstration, convey to the clinician their proactive and reactive strategies for dealing with the dysphagia. During the clinical evaluation, contributing and maintaining causes are determined by examination and by deductions that rule out the least likely causes and focus on those that are probable. Because feeding behaviors are among the earliest developing skills and are central to the child's well-being, the dysphagia may be the first symptom of a larger problem to demand attention, and medical consultations will inevitably occur later to determine the primary diagnosis and appropriate management. Alternatively, the clinical dysphagia evaluation may be initiated as part of a larger diagnostic workup. Its purposes are to describe the characteris-

Table 3–2 Consequences of Pediatric Feeding and Swallowing Disorders

Medical Issues
  Failure to thrive
  Pulmonary disorder
  Increased risk for choking
Behavioral Issues
  Prolonged and uncomfortable mealtime experiences
  Stressors in the parent-child relationship
Developmental Issues
  Failure to advance eating skills
  Drooling

tics of the dysphagia, particularly with reference to oral preparation of the bolus; pre-, intra- and post-prandial symptoms of respiratory, cardiac, and gastrointestinal perturbations; and behaviors associated with the meal. These observations are used to develop hypotheses as to the contributing and maintaining causes, which will be tested by further diagnostic evaluations and by the child's response to treatment. As in the adult clinical examination of dysphagia (CED), the pediatric CED includes examination of facial, oral, and pharyngeal anatomy for deformity and symptoms of paralysis; examination of oral mucosa, dentition, oral postural control, phonology, and voice; tests of reactivity of gag and velar reflexes; observations of control of oral secretions by spontaneous dry swallows; and observations of swallows elicited by bolus presentations. Table 3–3 summarizes the special features of the pediatric CED.

Special Features of the Pediatric Clinical Evaluation

History and Physical Examination. During the pediatric CED, additional history regarding developmental milestones for acquisition of feeding skills and adequacy of growth, including weight and height, is solicited. The examination includes inspection of the abdomen and thorax for adequacy of movements used to control breathing. The usual examination of gag, velar reflex, cough, and swallow is supplemented by tests for primitive oral reflexes, which are active during the first year of life in normal children and frequently persist into adulthood in individuals with early onset neurologic disorders (Sheppard, 1964; Sheppard & Mysak, 1984). The reflex examination provides an estimate of oral sensory and movement capabilities and impairments, which is most closely approximated by

---

Table 3–3 Special Features of the Pediatric Clinical Evaluation of Dysphagia

History
  Developmental milestones for eating skills
  Growth
Physical Examination
  Respiratory movements
  Primitive oral reflexes
  Non-nutritive suckling
Bolus Swallows
  Suckling
  Trials of bolus type and utensil sequenced by developmental expectations
Behaviors Associated with Eating
  State maintenance
  Tolerance of sensations and experiences associated with feeding tasks
  Acceptance of appropriate variety and quantity of foods

the localization of touch and range-of-movement tests that are often included in the adult clinical examination. In infants, examination of control of oral secretions at resting flow level and during the increased flow, which is stimulated by the oral inspection, is supplemented by observation of swallow during non-nutritive suckling (NNS). The rate of suckling and swallowing, and the movements and intraoral pressure adjustments that are seen in NNS are compared with nutritive suckling (Palmer, 1993).

Bolus Swallows. When examining elicited bolus swallows, the taste, viscosity, texture, and size of the test boluses; the selection of "utensil" for bolus delivery; and the child's independence in feeding are restricted to accommodate the child's current level of eating behavior, whether the child is NPO or PO, the child's performance expectations for age, and the child's experiences with food types and utensils. Presumptive levels of difficulty of bolus types for the normal child are: (1) resting level of salivary accumulation, (2) increased salivary flow in response to the oral examination, (3) nipple-fed liquid, (4) semi-solid puree, (5) pudding, consistency puree, (6) liquids from cup, (7) mashed, moist food, (8) crisp and soft chewable texture, (9) firmer chewable texture, (10) mixed, chewable texture, and (11) food that is fibrous and hard to chew. These are examined in order, with each subsequent test contingent on satisfactory management at the previous level. Biting is mastered before chewing. In each food category, small boluses are swallowed before larger ones. Appropriate oral and pharyngeal coordinations are mastered during dependent eating before self-feeding. In the child with dysphagia, some differences may alter the sequence of presentation. Spooned puree may be controlled better than liquid; thicker liquid may be controlled better than thin; and cup drinking may be easier than suckling. Table 3–4 summarizes levels of difficulty for bolus types and delivery of bolus.

When difficulties occur during early infancy, it often is assumed that bottle feeding will be more successful than breast feeding; however, this assumption has not been confirmed. Although there are fewer variables to control during bottle feeding and the results of a feeding are more readily apparent, clinical experiences suggest that resolution of suckling difficulties are frequently equally difficult during both breast and bottle feeding. Consideration of the difficulty of reception of bolus is, likewise, important when testing function with cup, straw, spoon, and fork and when determining the adequacy of the dual functions of self-feeding and oral management of bolus.

State and Other Behavioral Issues. It is important to determine any behavioral problems that are contributing to and maintaining the dysphagia. The first level of the analysis pertains to the child's "state" during feeding (Brazelton, 1973). A quiet, alert state with the child responsive to the cues that are relevant to the eating

Table 3-4 Presumptive Levels of Difficulty of Bolus Types and Bolus Delivery for the Normally Developing Child

> **Non-food Bolus**
>   Resting level of salivary flow
>   Stimulated salivary flow during non-nutritive suckling
>   Stimulated salivary flow during mouthing or oral examination
> **Food Bolus**
>   Nipple-fed liquid
>   Spoon-fed semi-solid puree
>   Spoon-fed pudding consistency puree
>   Liquids from cup
>   Spoon-fed mashed moist food
>   Finger-fed food that is crisp and soft to chew
>   Forked, firmer, chewable food
>   Mixed chewable textures
>   Food that is fibrous and hard to chew
> **Independence**
>   Dependent-feeding
>   Self-feeding
>   Bottle
>   Biscuit
>   Finger foods
>   Cup
>   Spoon

task is optimal for adequate intake, learning compensations, advancing skills, and avoiding conditioned aversions and phobias. As with adults, state variance, from somnolence to decompensation, should be noted. When the state is incompatible with good performance, efforts should be made to manage the behavioral difficulties and resolve the contributing issues.

Maintenance of the appropriate state for feeding and for advancing feeding skills is closely related to the child's tolerance for the sensations and experiences that are associated with eating. The child must become accustomed to eating in upright postures and sitting in a chair. Familiarity with variety of tastes, textures, viscosities, and bolus sizes must be established. Tolerance is acquired for the sensations associated with the variety of utensils used for bolus delivery and with the combined hand-mouth actions needed for self-feeding. And the intimate social interactions associated with feeding must be, at least, tolerable and, at best, reinforcing for the child (Sheppard, 1995).

Dowling (1980) reported on behavioral outcomes in a longitudinal study of infants who were tube-fed because of esophageal atresia. All the infants had limited experiences with oral feeding, independent food seeking, hunger-contingent satiation, and the usual caregiving interactions associated with feeding. The infants who demonstrated more undesirable effects had experienced gastrostomy feeding on predetermined schedules that were not contingent on expressions of hunger or arousal. They did not have the "sham oral feeding" routines that, when used with tube feeding, associate the experience of satiation with oral intake, and their mothers demonstrated attitudes of hopelessness or hostility in caring for a disabled child. These children experienced retardation in gross and fine motor coordination, and they had poorly developed interpersonal attachment, poorly developed interest in toys, diminished use of mouth for exploration, and, when oral feeding was initiated, lack of expression of hunger. These problems were diminished or absent in the children who experienced ordinary, good "mothering," and oral feeding of milk and solids administered during the gastrostomy feeding while the child was held in the mother's arms.

Rudolph (1994) discussed two categories of behavioral feeding disorder: (1) specific food aversions, usually linked to particular food tastes or textures; and (2) more generalized food aversions that restrict quantity of intake. He associates the former with temporary juxtaposition of feeding with aversive experiences, such as chemotherapy. He associates the latter with aspiration, choking, or pain occurring in proximity to feeding. Gastroesophageal reflux (GER) and visceral hyperalgesia have been suggested as similarly potent conditioners (Hyman, 1994). DiScipio and colleagues (1978) call this problem "traumatically conditioned dysphagia" when it persists in children whose dysphagia has resolved or has improved enough to permit the child to resume or advance oral feeding. Singer and colleagues (1991) note that children with chronic health problems are more prone to develop behavioral feeding disorders. Fifty-seven percent of a sample of children with cystic fibrosis who were older than 1 year reported feeding problems that, in some cases, were sufficient to cause malnutrition. Singer and colleagues attribute this to the special nature of the experiences between parent and child. The parents experienced increased personal and family stresses, and had a lower sense of parental competence; the child had more acute illness, fatigue, and separation from caregivers.

Instrumental Examination

If there are or have been symptoms of involvement of pharyngeal and/or esophageal phases of swallow that were of sufficient severity to be associated with nutritional or pulmonary problems, the clinical evaluation should be supplemented by instrumental evaluation. The purposes, as in the adult instrumental examination, are to rule out organic causes that could be treated; to determine the movement components of oral, pharyngeal, and esophageal phases of swallow; and to test the effectiveness of compensations for improving swallowing safety and efficiency. This testing is also appropriate in instances when initiation of oral feeding is advised for the child who has been NPO because of dysphagia and when the child is an oral feeder but is unable to maintain adequate nutrition. Instrumentation techniques that are useful in pediatrics are videofluoroscopy and related radiographic studies, ultrasound, nasopharyngeal endoscopy, pH probe, scintigraphy, and esophageal manometry (Arvedson & Rogers, 1993; Willging, 1994).

Videofluoroscopy and Related Radiographic Studies

Videofluoroscopy is the most frequently used technique in spite of the inherent difficulties in securing valid and reliable results from a child who may be apprehensive; resistant to oral intake, especially if the taste is unfamiliar; and used to more assistance than the radiology equipment will permit. The pediatric radiograph study is structured to accommodate the child's individual capabilities and preferences to a greater extent than the standard adult study (Logemann, 1993; Marquis & Pressman, 1995). Optimally, the prescription for the study includes both modified barium swallow (MBS) and upper gastrointestinal (UGI) studies, thus providing the option to examine bolus motility from lips to intestine. This latitude is useful especially for the child who, before the examination, cannot describe the symptoms that would localize the problem. In addition, the prevalence of GI complications is high in children and adults with developmental disability, and should be ruled out, if possible, when a swallowing study is performed (Laraya-Cuasay & Mikkilineni, 1995; Marquis & Pressman, 1995; Sheppard, Liou, Hochman, Laroia, & Langlois, 1988).

The positioning equipment used to stabilize the child during the study should provide the opportunity to observe ingestion in the typical mealtime gravitational positions and in alignments that may facilitate improved bolus motility. Special chairs and cervical collars are used to achieve these ends (Kramer, 1989; Marquis & Pressman, 1995; Woods, 1995). Familiar foods mixed with barium are provided to facilitate acceptance and optimum motor organization for ingestion (Gentile, 1987). Methods for bolus delivery vary depending on the child's prior experience, abilities, and willingness to ingest food. In some children, independent use of typical utensils (nipple bottle, straw, cup, spoon, and fingers) has been established and may be allowed during the radiology study. For these children, the clinician assists to regulate bolus size and rate of intake.

Many children, however, have difficulty with oral transport or refuse boluses that are delivered by typical utensils. These children tax the clinician's resourcefulness and flexibility. Marquis and Pressman (1995) describe strategies that are effective for these children. Two utensil adaptations that permit the clinician to control size of bolus and rate of bolus delivery, and facilitate or bypass oral preparation of the bolus are a nipple attached to a syringe by a length of flexible tubing and a syringe attached to a short piece of tubing. Both permit controlled placement of the bolus in the mouth. In the child who refuses oral intake, a nasogastric tube may be passed and, under radiologic guidance, withdrawn through the esophagus and into the pharynx as boluses are discharged. This procedure allows examination of gastric filling and emptying, esophageal motility, and pharyngeal swallow (Marquis & Pressman, 1995).

Ultrasonography

Ultrasonography is the preferred method for examining intra-oral coordinations for oral preparation and oral initiation phases of swallow in the infant and young child. During suckling, submental placement of the transducer allows simultaneous visualization of the nipple, tongue surface and subsurface musculature, hard and soft palate, hyoid, and the upper margin of the larynx in the sagittal plane (Weber, Woolridge, & Baum, 1986; Bosma, Hepburn, Josell, & Baker, 1990). The instrumentation also allows visualization in the coronal plane tongue of movement on the nipple with submental placement, and visualization in the transverse (transbuccal) plane of tongue movement on the nipple with buccal placement (Smith, Erenberg, Nowak, & Franken, 1985). Observation of vocal fold movement is achieved in the transverse plane with cervical placement. Doppler provides additional information regarding bolus flow. Capabilities for determining the occurrence of aspiration are limited; however, liquid flow through the glottis may be visualized in the transverse cervical plane using Doppler. Feeding can be observed in typical postural alignment, using typical foods and utensils. The instrumentation does not limit duration and frequency of observations in any way. Ultrasonography is particularly useful for testing the child who cannot tolerate videofluoroscopy, observing changes in function during the course of a meal, determining the immediate effectiveness of intervention strategies, and documenting the ongoing effects of treatment (Kenny, Casas, & McPherson, 1989; Casas, Kenny, & McPherson, 1994). Additionally, ultrasonography has been used for these purposes and for examining oral-pharyngeal movements and timing in older children and adults (Shawker, Sonies, Stone, & Baum, 1983; Sonies, Parent, Morrish, & Baum, 1988).

MANAGEMENT

Effective clinical management of the child with dysphagia arises from consideration of the effects of contributing causes on developing physiologic and social systems. Cooperation among the feeding specialist, the day-to-day caregivers, the educators, and the medical and allied health professionals who are attending to the significant psychological, motor, medical, surgical, dental, and nutritional needs of the child is optimal and may be essential for the child with a more complex and severe disorder (Rosenthal et al., 1995). Of utmost importance is the training of caregivers and educators to enable them to enhance the child's opportunities to habituate compensations, advance skills, and avoid habituation of maladaptive patterns.

Early Intervention

Timing of intervention is important. The best results are achieved when therapy begins at the onset of the disorder. Early attention to readiness before initiating or advancing oral feeding reduces the likelihood of secondary physiologic and psychological problems that may prolong habilation (Willging, 1994). Prompt attention to medical and dental needs is important to avoid their debilitating and traumatic effects. Otolaryngological, gastrointestinal, pulmonary, and maxillofacial disorders have been found to be potent conditioners of food refusal and feeding phobias. Early and ongoing attention to the nutritional needs of the child with dysphagia is warranted for maintaining good general health, growth, and ability to benefit from treatment interventions.

Procedures for Improving Feeding Skills and Swallowing

In pediatrics, the dysphagia therapy program includes advancing developmental skills and improving underlying movement competencies for acquisition of mature, safe, ingestion behaviors. Intervention may be indicated to develop the prescriptive feeding procedures for optimum nutrition, safety, and efficiency and to improve underlying competencies for the task components of swallow. A child may need to be trained regarding the oral preparatory milestones of suckling, spoon feeding, cup drinking, chewing, self-feeding, and the task components that are involved in these skills. These task components include reception, anterior and posterior containment, oral manipulation, and formation of the bolus. In addition, development of oral initiation skills for propelling larger and more viscous boluses and for coordinating breathing with oral preparation of the bolus and swallowing may require training. Improving the psychosocial aspects of feeding regarding food acceptance and compliance during meals is important in pediatric dysphagia therapy. Thus, behavior modification, operant conditioning, and cognitive behavioral approaches are used more frequently (DiScipio et al., 1978; Singer, Ambuel, Wade, & Jaffe, 1992). There is generally less reliance on didactic instruction in pediatrics and more frequent use of compensatory strategies, grading of task difficulty, assisted exercise, and repetitive and rhythmic exercise routines to provide functional contexts in which more adequate and advanced feeding and swallowing may be practiced (Sheppard, 1995).

CASE STUDIES

Case histories that illustrate typical management strategies for problems in children with dysphagia are presented. In case 1, suckling problems are resolved in a premature infant with birth complications. Case 2 describes a young, developmentally disabled child with a complex medical history who makes a successful transition from tube to oral feeding. In case 3, a child with cerebral palsy, and medical and developmental disorders is managed with consideration for her disability and for her family's decisions regarding her care.

Case 1

A.R. was delivered by Caesarean section at 37 weeks gestation after spontaneous onset of labor. She weighed 5 lbs, 13 oz. Her mother was medicated for hypertension during pregnancy. Birth complications were meconium aspiration and sepsis. A.R. was intubated, suctioned, and placed on continuous positive airway pressure (CPAP). She was NPO for 3 days, accepted 20 cc nipple feeds on day 4, and was discharged with her mother on day 5. Breast feeding, initiated on day 5 at home, was unsuccessful. Typically, the child latched and suckled, but came off the nipple crying soon after the flow began. Bottle feeding was problematic with slow and limited intake, ranging from 1 to 4 oz. Nourishment was provided with combination of breast- and bottle-feeding with breast milk. Feeding occurred every 2 hours; weight gain was slow; there were infrequent stools; and the child was agitated and did not calm after feeding. Regurgitation was not considered to be excessive, and the infant's respiratory condition was stable. The mother wanted to feed by breast if possible. The child was referred by her pediatrician for consultations by lactation and feeding specialists at 4 weeks old because of failing nutrition and persistent difficulties with feeding.

Significant clinical findings included apprehensiveness during oral digital examination and when initiating suckling, She reacted by body stiffening, tongue posturing to avoid entry, and gagging. Bursts of "transitional stage" suckling (Palmer, 1993) occurred, during which she held her breath for three to five suckle-swallows. These behaviors were associated with crying and breaking away from nipple. There was diminished productivity of suckling during the feeding. The child remained alert during feeding. Non-nutritive suckling and single bolus swallows were competent.

The clinical impression was dysphagia with involvement in oral initiation of swallow. Contributing causes were: (1) traumatic effects of early intubation, suctioning, and NPO status; (2) immature suckling pattern, characterized by episodic incoordination of breathing and suckle-swallow; and (3) presumptive GI discomfort, occurring as feeding progressed and associated with infrequent stools.

The management plan was to provide feeding predominantly by bottle with short breast feeding twice daily. Mother was instructed to position the infant securely, supported close to her body. She was instructed to bottle feed with the child resting on right side or more upright than recumbent, and to pace the infant's suckling and breathing by removing her from the nipple when she began to hold her breath during more than two suckle-swallow cycles. A finger or pacifier was to replace the nipple in the infant's mouth for a few breath cycles before feeding resumed. It was suggested that breast feeding be initiated after pumping the breast to partially empty it. Between feedings, the mother was to engage in pleasant vocal interaction and oral digital play with the infant with finger dipped in breast milk. The infant was allowed to signal her hunger before a feeding was initiated. As tolerance for breast improved, bottle feeding would be reduced gradually and feeding off of a fuller breast initiated. The mother was urged to consult with the pediatrician regarding management for the infrequent stools.

At 8 weeks old, A.R. was feeding well at the breast, weight gain was satisfactory, and she was feeding on demand at approximately 4-hour intervals.

Case 2

A.S. is a 2-year-old child with diagnosis of 17p- syndrome with hypotonia, developmental delay, defective vision, and dysphagia. She had a gastrostomy at 1 month because of difficulty feeding. She has a history of vocal stridor, severe gastroesophageal reflux (GER) with copious vomiting and coughing during gastrostomy tube (GT) feeding until 1 year. She experienced one episode of viral pneumonia 3 months before evaluation, but respiratory health had been good otherwise. Growth had been satisfactory. Modified barium swallow (MBS) study conducted at 5 months old revealed laryngeal penetration (i.e., passage of the bolus into the laryngeal vestibule) on thin liquids, but no aspiration (i.e., penetration of the bolus below the vocal folds). A program for implementing the transition from tube to oral feeding was begun at that time using pureed food. At the time of this evaluation, intake was limited to pureed, baby food fruits or vegetables, given twice daily in 1- to 2-oz portions. This re-evaluation by a tertiary care dysphagia team was initiated by her mother because of limited progress with oral feeding.

Significant clinical findings were: (1) piecemeal swallowing of spooned bolus; (2) poorly coordinated breathing and swallowing while eating pureed food; (3) increased respiratory rate after a few tastes followed by refusal to continue accepting boluses; (4) slightly wet breath sounds after bolus swallows; and (5) apparent anxiety during bolus swallows and during non-nutritive mouthing tasks. Modified barium swallow study revealed safe bolus swallows on puree and thin liquid with no evidence of laryngeal penetration or tracheal aspiration. Radiograph observations confirmed that bolus size was restricted by piecemeal delivery of the bolus into the pharynx, and that swallows became less organized as feeding progressed. No pharyngeal stasis was seen on radiograph for liquid or puree. Nutritional evaluation found A.S. to be heavier than the desired weight for height.

The clinical impression was dysphagia with impairment in oral preparation, oral initiation, and pharyngeal phases of swallowing. Contributing causes were: (1) traumatically conditioned effects of GER; and (2) inadequate amount of practice for acquisition of the skills needed for oral feeding.

A management plan was developed to increase acceptance of food from spoon and cup. The parent was referred back to the physical therapist for modifications of the child's feeding chair to improve ability to actively move onto the spoon and cup as they were brought to her mouth. The immediate objectives for therapeutic feeding were: (1) to improve tolerance for cup, spoon, and the taste of two foods— one for spoon and one for cup; (2) to habituate active movement onto cup and spoon; and (3) to increase amount and rate of intake. A behavior modification program was developed in cooperation with the parent which provided for two short, daily, practice sessions. A limited number of tastes from cup and spoon would be offered. There would be consistent positive reinforcement after each taste regardless of whether it was swallowed. The number of tastes, size of bolus, and, eventually, type of foods would be increased weekly (Sheppard, 1995). The number of sessions with the feeding therapist were to be increased for the short term until the program was established. Subsequent adjustments in GT and oral feeding would be made as the child progressed. The dietician recommended reduction in calories in the GT feeding to allow height to catch up with weight.

At 2 years, 9 months, oral intake had increased sufficiently for gastrostomy tube feeding to be discontinued. At 2 years, 10 months, the child was doing well on oral feeding and a program to advance eating skills was initiated.

Case 3

V.E. is a 14-year, 3-month-old child with diagnoses of static encephalopathy with microcephaly, cerebral palsy spastic quadriplegia, profound mental retardation, alternating exotropia, scoliosis, seizure disorder, and dysphagia. She had had hip adductor release surgery and selective posterior rhizotomy. She is medicated for seizures with Tegretol and Depakote but continues to have modified complex partial seizures many times each day. She is reported to have asthma that is triggered by upper respiratory infection and is given Ventolin orally as needed for wheezing. She had many episodes of pneumonia when younger, with the most recent episode occurring 1 year ago. She is given Senokot and glycerine suppositories for constipation. She was medicated with Reglan for a trial period, which the family found to be helpful. The medication was discontinued because of concern about side effects. Recently, she had been referred to a gastroenterologist but the appointment has not yet been made. Weight for height is below the fifth percentile. Presently, she is fed a pureed table food diet by spoon and liquids by cup. She is fed in another's lap or in an adaptive seat. Meals are prolonged at 30 to 60 minutes. She sounds congested during meals. Intake is limited and there may be crying after eating. V.E. was referred to the tertiary care dysphagia team because of coughing and gagging associated with eating. The referral was initiated by her school staff. Her mother agreed to the comprehensive evaluation providing that the recommendations would focus on improving oral feeding.

Significant clinical findings were: (1) special chair and assistance needed to stabilize head-neck and thorax in sitting position during feeding; (2) small mandible and marked distoclusion; (3) oral secretions that pooled in the mouth and in oral pharynx; (4) reduced mouth opening and tongue blocking were used to control the timing of bolus entry and size of bolus; (5) slow oral transport of bolus; (6) multiple swallows to clear each bolus; and (7) congested breath sounds during and after feeding. The dietician's evaluation found the child's intake to be 861 calories per day, approximately 50% of her daily needs. Modified barium swallow study revealed poor posterior containment of the bolus before initiating swallow. Filling of the pyriform sinuses before the swallow and stasis in valleculae and pyriform sinuses after the swallow were seen with multiple swallows used to clear each bolus from the pharynx. With pureed bolus, laryngeal penetration and tracheal aspiration occurred after the swallow. With liquid bolus, laryngeal penetration with trace tracheal aspiration was noted after the swallow. Pharyngeal contraction was diminished and ineffectual on all swallows. There was no coughing or gagging. Frontal chest radiograph obtained after examination revealed barium in the left lower lobe bronchi.

The clinical impression was severe dysphagia with involvement in oral preparatory, oral initiation, and pharyngeal phases of swallow. Contributing causes were static encephalopathy, cerebral palsy, breakthrough seizures, and oral and thoracic skeletal deformities. There was severe malnutrition and reactive airway disease.

The mother was counseled regarding the results of the evaluation. A management plan for continued oral feeding was devised and it was recommended that a pediatric gastroenterologist be consulted for further evaluation and discussion of the best means of feeding. Oral feeding should occur while the child is sitting in a chair to provide appropriate assistance to stabilize the head and neck. Diet viscosity should be moderated to ease oral and pharyngeal transport. Thin pudding solids and thick liquids were recommended. High-calorie, full-nutrient supplements should be provided. The child should be rested before feeding to minimize fatigue. Bolus size should be limited to one-half teaspoon. Feeding time should be limited to 30 minutes with additional feedings provided as needed to increase intake. It was suggested that nebulized Proventil might be more effective and that the child might benefit from "chest physical therapy" exercise on a regular basis. An oral exercise program was recommended with the goals of improving or maintaining adequate swallowing for oral secretions and for oral feeding if this type of feeding was to continue.

During the team discussion, it was agreed that non-oral feeding would be best from a respiratory and nutrition perspective. Concerns were expressed regarding the child's suitability for surgery, her history of reflux, and the possibility of increased management problems with weight gain. A summary of the team discussion was included in the report.

At 14 years, 9 months, V.E. underwent gastrostomy and Nissan fundoplication. Surgery was successful and nutrition and respiratory health have continued to improve.

CONCLUSION

Feeding behaviors are among the earliest developing voluntary behaviors in infants. Their relationship to parent-child interactions, psychosocial development, acquisition of developing oral motor skills, nutrition, and respiratory health are well recognized. Dysphagia occurs as a complication in infants and children with a variety of medical and developmental disorders. Early and comprehensive management of dysphagia is important to minimize the wide ranging primary and secondary medical and developmental consequences that may occur.

REFERENCES

Als, H. (1986). A synactive model of neonatal behavioral organization: Development in the premature infant and for support of infants and parents in the neonatal intensive care environment. *Physical and Occupational Therapy in Pediatrics, 6,* 3–53.

Arvedson, J.C., & Rogers, B.T. (1993). Pediatric swallowing and feeding disorders. *Journal of Medical Speech-Language Pathology, 1* (4), 203–221.

Brazelton, T.B. (1973). Neonatal behavioral assessment scale: clinics in developmental medicine, number 50. *Spastics International Medical Publications.* Philadelphia: J.B. Lippincott.

Bazyk, S. (1990). Factors associated with the transition to oral feeding in infants fed by nasogastric tubes. *The American Journal of Occupational Therapy, 44* (12), 1070–1078.

Bosma, J.F. (1988). Functional anatomy of the upper airway during development. In O.P. Mathew & G. Sant'Ambrogio (Eds.), *Respiratory function of the upper airway* (pp. 47–86). New York: Marcel Dekker.

Bosma, J.F., Hepburn, L.G., Josell, S.D., & Baker, K. (1990). Ultrasound demonstration of tongue motions during suckle feeding. *Developmental Medicine and Child Neurology, 32,* 223–229.

Casas, M.D., Kenny, D.J., & McPherson, K.A. (1994). Swallowing ventilation interactions during oral swallow in normal children and children with cerebral palsy. *Dysphagia, 9,* 40–46.

DiScipio, W., Kaslon, K., & Ruben, R. (1978). Traumatically acquired conditioned dysphagia in children. *Annals of Otology, Rhinology, and Laryngology, 87*(4 Pt. 1), 509–514.

Dowling, S. (1980). Going forth to meet the environment: A developmental study of seven infants with esophageal atresia. *Psychosomatic Medicine, 42*(1:II, supplement 1980), 153–161.

Fleisher, D.R. (1994). Functional vomiting disorders in infancy: Innocent vomiting, nervous vomiting, and infant rumination syndrome. *Journal of Pediatrics, 125*(6 Pt. 2), S84–S93.

Gentile, A.M. (1987). Skill acquisition: Action, movement and neuromotor processes. In J.H. Carr & R.B. Shepherd (Eds.), *Movement sciences: Foundations for physical therapy in rehabilitation.* Gaithersburg, MD: Aspen Publishers.

Gisel, E.G. (1991). Effect of food texture on the development of chewing in children between six months and two years of age. *Developmental Medicine and Child Neurology, 33*, 69–79.

Handleman, J. (1995). Raising a child with developmental disability. In S. Rosenthal, J.J. Sheppard, & M. Lotze (Eds.), *Dysphagia and the child with developmental disabilities: Medical, clinical and family interventions.* San Diego, CA: Singular Publishing Group.

Hyman, P.E. (1994). Gastroesophageal reflux: One reason why baby won't eat. *Journal of Pediatrics, 125*(6 Pt. 2), S103–S109.

Illingworth, R.S., & Lister, J. (1964). The critical or sensitive period with special reference to feeding problems in infants and children. *Journal of Pediatrics, 65*, 836–848.

Ingram, T.T. (1962). Clinical significance of the infantile feeding reflexes. *Developmental Medicine and Child Neurology, 4*, 159–169.

Kenny, D.J., Casas, M.D., & McPherson, K.A. (1989). Correlation of ultrasound imaging of oral swallow with ventilatory alterations in cerebral palsied and normal children. *Dysphagia, 4*, 16–28.

Kramer, S.S. (1989). Radiologic examination of the swallowing impaired child. *Dysphagia, 3*, 117–125.

Laraya-Cuasay, L., & Mikkilineni, S. (1995). Respiratory conditions and care. In S. Rosenthal, J.J. Sheppard, & M. Lotze (Eds.), *Dysphagia and the child with developmental disabilities: Medical, clinical, and family interventions.* San Diego, CA: Singular Publishing Group.

Logemann, J.A. (1993). *Manual for the videofluorographic study of swallowing* (2nd ed.). Austin, TX: Pro-Ed.

Marquis, J., & Pressman, H. (1995). Radiologic assessment of pediatric swallowing. In S. Rosenthal, J.J. Sheppard, & M. Lotze (Eds.), *Dysphagia and the child with developmental disabilities: Medical, clinical and family interventions.* San Diego, CA: Singular Publishing Group.

Mascarenhas, M.R., & Dadhania, J. (1995). Gastrointestinal problems. In S. Rosenthal, J.J. Sheppard, & M. Lotze (Eds.), *Dysphagia and the child with developmental disabilities: Medical, clinical and family interventions.* San Diego, CA: Singular Publishing Group.

Newman, L.A., Cleveland, R.H., Blickman, J.G., Hillman, R.E., & Jaramillo, D. (1991). Video-fluoroscopic analysis of the infant swallow. *Investigative Radiology, 26*, 870–873.

Palmer, M.M. (1993). Identification and management of the transitional suck pattern in premature infants. *Journal of Perinatal and Neonatal Nursing, 7* (1), 66–75.

Rosenthal, S., Sheppard, J.J., & Lotze, M. (1995). *Dysphagia in the child with developmental disabilities, Medical: clinical and family interventions.* San Diego, CA: Singular Publishing Group.

Rubin, I.L., & Crocker, A.C. (1989). *Developmental disabilities, delivery of medical care for children and adults.* Philadelphia: Lea & Febiger.

Rudolph, C.D. (1994). Feeding disorders in infants and children. *Journal of Pediatrics, 125*(6 Pt. 2), S116–S124.

Shawker, T.H., Sonies, B., Stone, M., & Baum, B.J. (1983). Real-time ultrasound visualization of tongue movement during swallowing. *Journal of Clinical Ultrasound, 11*, 485–490.

Sheppard, J.J. (1964). Cranio-oropharyngeal motor patterns in dysarthria associated with cerebral palsy. *Journal of Speech and Hearing Research, 7,* 373–380.

Sheppard, J.J. (1995). Clinical evaluation and treatment. In S. Rosenthal, J.J. Sheppard, & M. Lotze (Eds.), *Dysphagia and the child with developmental disabilities: Medical, clinical and family interventions.* San Diego, CA: Singular Publishing Group.

Sheppard, J.J., Liou, J., Hochman, R., Laroia, S., & Langlois, D. (1988). Nutritional correlates of dysphagia in individuals institutionalized with mental retardation. *Dysphagia, 3,* 85–89.

Sheppard, J.J., & Mysak, E.D. (1984). Ontogeny of infantile oral reflexes and emerging chewing. *Child Development, 55,* 831–843.

Sheppard, J.J., & Pressman, H. (1988). Dysphagia in infantile cortical hyperostosis (Caffey's Disease): A case study. *Developmental Medicine Child Neurology, 30,* 108–114.

Singer, L. (1990). When a sick child won't—or can't—eat. *Contemporary Pediatrics, December,* 60–76.

Singer, L.T., Ambuel, B., Wade, S., & Jaffe, A.C. (1992). Cognitive-behavioral treatment of health-impairing food phobias in children. *Journal of the American Academy of Child Adolescent Psychiatry, 31* (5), 847–852.

Singer, L.T., Nofer, J.A., Benson-Szekely, L.J., & Brooks, L.J. (1991). Behavioral assessment and management of food refusal in children with cystic fibrosis. *Developmental and Behavioral Pediatrics, 12* (2), 115–120.

Smith, W.L., Erenberg, A., Nowak, A., & Franken, E.A. (1985). Physiology of sucking in the normal term infant using real time US. *Radiology, 156,* 379–381.

Sonies, B.C., & Kahane, J. (1992a, February). *Possible effects of anatomical age-related change of epiglottis and hyoid bone on swallowing: In vivo, in vitro comparisons.* Presented at Effects on Quality of Life Conference, National Institutes of Health National Institutes of Aging, Washington, DC.

Sonies, B.C., & Kahane, J. (1992b, November). *Aging and swallowing: Effects of changes of hyoid and epiglottis.* Presented at American Speech-Language-Hearing Association Convention, San Antonio, TX.

Sonies, B.C., Parent, B.S., Morrish, K., & Baum, B.J. (1988). Durational aspects of the oral-pharyngeal phase of swallow in normal adults. *Dysphagia, 3,* 1–10.

Stolovitz, P., & Gisel, E.G. (1991). Circumoral movements in response to three different food textures in children 6-months to 2-years of age. *Dysphagia, 6* (1), 17–25.

Stroh, K., Robinson, T., & Stroh, G. (1986). A therapeutic feeding programme I: Theory and practice of feeding. *Developmental Medicine and Child Neurology, 28* (1), 3–10.

Weber, F., Woolridge, M.W., & Baum, J.D. (1986). An ultrasonographic study of the organization of sucking and swallowing by newborn infants. *Developmental Medicine and Child Neurology, 28,* 19–24.

Willging, J.P. (1994). Swallowing disorders in children. *Current Science, 2,* 504–507.

Woods, E.K. (1995). The influence of posture and positioning on oral motor development and dysphagia. In S. Rosenthal, J.J. Sheppard, & M. Lotze (Eds.), *Dysphagia and the child with developmental disabilities: Medical, clinical and family interventions.* San Diego, CA: Singular Publishing Group.

PART II

External Issues That Impact Treatment

CHAPTER 4

Legal Implications in Dysphagia Practice

Paula C. Ohliger

Our society has become increasingly litigious over the past 20 years. Health care providers have felt the pressure associated with and fear of being named in a lawsuit. Speech and language pathologists who are involved in the treatment of dysphagia express concern about the potential for liability related to such treatment. Potential risks arise not only from the speech pathologist's relationship with the patient, but also with the physician, the patient's family, and third party payers. To decrease the risk of lawsuits, it is important to understand what constitutes professional negligence and how to protect oneself from such liability.

This chapter reviews the elements that must be present for a health care professional to be found liable for professional negligence. It then discusses strategies available to the speech and language pathologist that may minimize the risks of such liability.

THE ELEMENTS OF MALPRACTICE—PROFESSIONAL NEGLIGENCE

Professional negligence is the primary legal cause of action likely to be brought against a health professional in a lawsuit for medical malpractice. To establish negligence, whether involving a health care provider or any other individual, a plaintiff must prove several elements. If any element is absent, the health care provider is not liable for negligence.

Note: This chapter is written with the understanding that the author is not engaged in rendering legal or other professional services. If legal or other expert assistance is required, the services of a competent professional should be sought. Nothing in this chapter is intended to create an attorney/client relationship as a result of the information provided herein.

The first element a plaintiff must demonstrate is the presence of a duty of care. The second element is a breach of the duty of care. The third element is foreseeable harm. The last element is "proximate causation."

Existence of a Duty of Care

The plaintiff must demonstrate that the health care provider had a duty of care in relation to a patient. Whether a duty of care exists depends on a variety of factors related to the relationship between individuals. A "special relationship" must exist between two individuals to impose a duty of care upon one to protect the other against harm.

A health care provider has a legal duty to protect others, but not in all situations. For example, health care professionals are under no legal obligation to save the life of a stranger, even if they could. Moreover, health care providers are under no legal duty to render professional services to every individual who seeks to engage them.[1] The mutual agreement between the patient and the health care professional creates the provider/patient relationship and imposes a duty on the health care provider to protect the patient from foreseeable harm.

The Standard of Care

The parameters of a health care provider's duty are defined by the standard of care that health care providers must follow. Generally, that duty is expressed as the duty to exercise "the reasonable degree of skill, knowledge, and care ordinarily possessed and exercised by members of the same profession under the same or similar circumstances."[2] The exact standard varies according to the particular facts of a situation. In the past, the phrase "same or similar circumstances" applied to the diagnosis and treatment methods used by a health care provider in the same locale or community. Thus, practitioners in a rural area were not necessarily expected to follow the same standard of care as those in larger urban areas. Today, with modern methods of communication and ease of access to information, a health care provider's duty of care is no longer fulfilled merely by using the treatment techniques available in his or her own region. Courts generally use a national standard of care rather than that of a local community. The true test is what a *reasonable* health care provider would do under the same or similar circumstances.

Health care providers are not to be held liable for negligence merely because their treatment was not successful.[3] In the absence of an expressed contract to that effect, health care providers do not warrant cures or guarantee the results of their services.[4] Thus, the mere fact that treatment results in negative, unforeseeable, or rare consequences does not mean that the health care provider is negligent. Moreover, a charge of malpractice may be disproved by evidence that, under similar circumstances, a patient might have suffered the same harm even if due care were exercised, or that injury invariably occurs in a certain number of cases of that kind.[5]

Health care providers are not omniscient or capable of knowing invariably that their professional acts will achieve a desired result. They are responsible only when it is established that they did not act with the knowledge or foresight a reasonably skillful and experienced practitioner would have demonstrated under the same or similar circumstances.[6] Nor does the law require that every health care provider have the skill of the most highly acclaimed expert in his or her field.[7] The health care provider must have only the reasonable skill and knowledge required of practitioners generally, unless the particular specialty requires a higher degree of knowledge.[8] Moreover, mere errors in judgment are not grounds for liability unless the skill and judgment used by the health care provider falls below the standard of care.[9] However, it is no defense that a health care provider used his or her best judgment if such judgment falls below the standard that would have been set by a reasonable practitioner under the same circumstances. In general, the practitioner who has and uses the degree of skill and knowledge required under the circumstances will not be liable for negligence.

The law recognizes that even the most skillful members of a profession may differ in what is considered "reasonable under the circumstances." The standard of care usually requires that a health care provider use recognized and approved methods of treatment. It is not necessary that a particular treatment be one chosen by the majority of health care providers. It is sufficient that a respectable minority of health care providers approve the treatment selected.[10] The mere fact that there is a difference of medical opinion concerning the desirability of one particular medical procedure over another does not establish that the use of one over the other is negligent.[11] Thus, the standard of care requires a health care provider to do only what is reasonable under the circumstances. Health care providers do not have to guarantee results, avoid errors in judgment, or use a particular treatment, as long as they use the skill and knowledge a reasonable practitioner would use.

Once the standard of care is established, the next question is whether the health care provider has met that standard. Did the health care provider do what a reasonable health care provider would do in the same or similar circumstances? Alternatively, did the health care provider fail to do something that should have been done? The answer to these questions depends on the specific facts of each case.

Foreseeable Harm

The second element of negligence is foreseeable harm. Even though a health care provider may have breached the standard of care, he or she will not be liable for negligence unless some kind of harm results from the breach. Even if the health care provider acted in the most unprofessional manner, if a patient does not suffer any harm or injury, the health care provider will not be liable for negligence. Moreover, the harm must be foreseeable. If the harm could not reasonably have been foreseen or anticipated, then negligence did not occur.

For example, imagine the following scenario. A speech and language pathologist is treating a child who has difficulty feeding himself because of underdeveloped oral reflexes and primitive motor responses. The child needs constant supervision by the therapist during feeding training. The speech pathologist leaves the child unsupervised for a few minutes while the child is eating. The child suffers no harm during the time he is left unsupervised. The speech pathologist's action of leaving the child unattended might be considered a breach of the standard of care because a reasonable clinician might not have left the child unsupervised. However, because no harm resulted, no negligence is present. If the child had aspirated while unsupervised, then the clinician may be liable for professional negligence if the clinician's actions are deemed to be below the standard of care.

The mere presence of harm, however, does not always indicate negligence. The harm must have been foreseeable. This means that a reasonable speech pathologist would have foreseen the type of harm that resulted from his or her actions. If a reasonable clinician could not have foreseen that harm would have resulted from his or her actions, or if the specific type of harm that resulted was not reasonably foreseeable, then there is no liability for negligence. For example, a speech pathologist's evaluation of a patient reveals that the patient has difficulty swallowing most liquids except for thick liquids. The speech pathologist recommends that the patient eat pureed foods and thick liquids only with supervision. The speech pathologist gives the patient a glass of water then leaves the patient unsupervised. The patient aspirates. The speech pathologist could be liable for negligence because it is reasonably foreseeable that a patient who cannot swallow thin liquids and requires supervision during feeding could aspirate if left unattended with a glass of water. Assuming that the action of leaving the patient unattended falls below the standard of care, the speech pathologist may be found liable for negligence.

Harm that is unforeseeable generally does not result in a finding of negligence. For example, in the situation described previously in which the child required supervision during feeding, assume that the speech pathologist leaves the child unattended. If the family dog comes into the room and bites the child while the speech pathologist is absent, the speech pathologist probably would not be liable for the injury. It is not reasonably foreseeable that leaving a patient with a swallowing problem unattended during feeding training would result in a dog bite. Although one might argue that the harm would not have happened if the speech pathologist had been in attendance, the dog bite is not the type of harm one would reasonably foresee happening. It this case, the unforeseeability of the harm would be a defense to the speech pathologist's negligent behavior.

Causation

The third element of negligence is causation. Even if a speech pathologist's actions fall below the standard of care, and even if the harm is foreseeable, there must be a "causal relationship" between the actions of the health care provider and the resulting harm. Causation involves two elements. The clinician's actions must be the "cause in fact" of the injury and the "proximate cause" of the injury.[12]

The first element of causation is "cause in fact." This element requires an injured party to demonstrate that the health care provider's actions contributed in some way to the injury so that "but for" the health care provider's actions, the injury would not have happened.[13] If the injury would have happened anyway, whether or not the health care provider's actions or omissions fell below the standard of care, then the actions are not a "cause in fact" and no legal cause exists.[14] For example, in the scenario described previously, the patient cannot swallow any foods except pureed foods or thick liquids. Imagine that the speech pathologist gives the patient a glass of water and the patient aspirates. "But for" the action of the speech pathologist, the patient would not have aspirated. Therefore, the actions of the speech pathologist are the "cause in fact" of the patient's harm. Because aspiration is a reasonably foreseeable result of the speech pathologist's actions, the speech pathologist would be liable for negligence, assuming that the speech pathologist's actions fell below the standard of care.

Occasionally, it may be difficult to determine if the harm would not have happened "but for" the health care provider's actions, for example in cases in which other actions or individuals are involved. In those cases, courts will consider whether the clinician's actions were such a "substantial factor" in producing the harm that a reasonable person would regard those actions as a cause of the harm.[15] For example, a speech pathologist's evaluation reveals that a patient needs supervision during feeding, but can be supervised by a nurse's aide. The speech pathologist leaves detailed written instructions for the aide, who is new to this particular hospital unit. The speech pathologist has never met the aide. The aide misunderstands some of the instructions and rushes the patient through the meal. The patient aspirates. Two actions are involved in the harm here: (1) the aide's failure to follow the clinician's instructions, and (2) the speech pathologist's failure to properly instruct the aide. In this case, the clinician's actions are likely to be a "substantial factor" in causing the harm because a reasonable person would likely regard them as a cause. Thus, the clinician's actions would be a "cause in fact" of the harm, even though another person's actions also "caused" the harm. Assuming all of the other elements of negligence are present, the clinician likely would be liable for negligence.

The second element involved in causation is "proximate cause." The rules of proximate causation are elusive and have been the subject of continued debate by legal experts and the courts. The doctrine of proximate causation serves to relieve an individual of liability even though his or her conduct is a "cause in fact" of an injury, if it would be considered "unjust" to hold him or her legally responsible.[16] The proximate cause doctrine limits liability because of the manner in which an injury occurred.[17] For example, when an intervening act is not reasonably foreseeable, the clinician's conduct is not deemed the "proximate cause" of the injury. The question is whether a person whose actions fall below the standard of care should be held liable for all of the consequences of those actions.

For example, in the previous scenario concerning the nurse's aide, imagine that the aide leaves the patient unattended even though the aide was instructed not to do so. During that period, the family comes in and takes the patient down the hall in the wheelchair. A nurse comes along and takes the patient to the bathroom. The nurse gives the patient a glass of water and the patient aspirates. In this case, there are several intervening events between the clinician's actions and the harm to the patient. The question in simple terms is whether these intervening acts were reasonably foreseeable by the clinician. It appears unlikely in this case that these actions were foreseeable even though the harm was of the type that was foreseeable. This is a complex area of the law. The main point to understand is that speech pathologists will not always be responsible for all consequences of their actions if imposing liability would be unjust under the circumstances.

The examples discussed previously show the application of the rules of causation in simple situations. As the number of factors increases, the analysis of liability becomes more complex. These general principles and examples are meant to be guidelines only. In general, if the actions or omissions of a speech pathologist fall below the standard of care and if such actions or omissions cause harm that was foreseeable, and thus was preventable, then the speech pathologist may be liable for professional negligence. However, if the actions do not fall below the standard of care, if no harm results, if the harm was not foreseeable, or if the actions did not cause the harm, either in fact or proximately, then no liability results.

PRACTICAL APPLICATIONS

Concerns about professional negligence arise from the speech pathologist's relationship with the patient. However, concerns arise in other areas as well. For example, a key area of concern is the relationship between the speech pathologist and the patient's family. Because dysphagia affects a basic activity of daily living, treatment often requires the hands-on assistance and cooperation of the family to be successful. This close interaction between the clinician and the patient's family can be the source of potential liability.

A second area of concern is the speech pathologist's relationship with the patient's physician. The clinician and the physician may differ in their opinions about a patient's treatment. This difference raises concerns about the speech pathologist's legal duty to the patient. In addition, the family often will attempt to influence the treating physician to order treatment with which the speech pathologist disagrees. This places the speech pathologist in a difficult position and again raises questions about the speech pathologist's legal and ethical duties to the patient.

A final area of concern arises in relation to decisions of third party payers. The question here is, "What are the legal duties and malpractice risks for the speech pathologist if a payer denies authorization for treatment that, in the speech pathologist's opinion, is medically necessary?"

A speech pathologist can follow certain guidelines that may help to decrease the risk of malpractice liability in relation to these three areas of concern. These guidelines are based on an application of the rules and elements of professional negligence.

The Relationship with the Family

Problems with families can take two different forms. First, a family might decline all treatment, assuming the family has the right to control the patient's health care decisions. Alternatively, the family might insist on a treatment that the speech pathologist believes is unsafe or inappropriate. The speech pathologist's actions must meet the standard of care (i.e., the speech pathologist must use the skill and knowledge that a reasonable speech pathologist would use under the same or similar circumstances). The question in these cases is, "What is reasonable under the circumstances?"

When a family declines treatment, the clinician should remember that, in many states, the family has the right to do so if they have the legal right to control the patient's health care decisions.[18] Consequently, the speech pathologist could accept the family's decision without incurring liability.[19] However, the speech pathologist should explain the treatment options and instruct the family and patient in the consequences of refusing treatment. If the family still declines, then the speech pathologist probably has done all that a reasonable clinician in the same position would do. The speech pathologist does not need to force a patient or family to follow a particular treatment decision.

If a speech pathologist has a difference of opinion with a patient's family or if the family is pressuring the speech pathologist to treat the patient in a manner that the speech pathologist believes is unsafe and/or inappropriate, the speech pathologist's first obligation is to keep the patient safe. Safety is key, especially with dysphagia patients for whom the negative consequences of improper treatment can be grave. Even if the speech pathologist, under pressure from the family, uses a treatment method that the speech pathologist believes may not be optimally safe (which may not necessarily be a "negligent" decision), the speech pathologist must ensure that the patient and the environment are as safe as reasonably possible under the circumstances.

In addition, it is essential that speech pathologists document all pertinent information clearly and completely. Documentation is the speech pathologist's primary defense tool. The patient's medical chart is the key evidence that will show what the speech pathologist did and why. Clear, complete, and competent documentation is essential to minimize malpractice liability. Documentation regarding family interactions should include not only the speech pathologist's clinical evaluation and treatment plan, but also the following information:

1. Document discussions with the family regarding treatment options and the family's reactions to those options. Disclose to the family the risks involved in all treatment options, including the family's desired options. Document the risks and the disclosure, as well as the family's choice to decline treatment and their reasons for declining or desiring certain treatment. Document the family's understanding of the risks involved in all these options.
2. Document instructions given to the family, including specific safety precautions. (Instructions should be written and included in the medical record.) Document the family's response to the instructions. Did the family understand the reasoning behind the instructions? Do they need further instructions or training?
3. Document recommendations and clinical opinions about treatment options, including safety concerns regarding the various treatment choices.
4. Document physician conferences concerning treatment options, family choices, and pressures. Include the physician's response to the family's concerns. Is the physician leaning toward the family's choices even though these choices are inappropriate? Document any differences of opinion with the physician.

There may be other issues and subjects that should be included in the patient's medical record as well. The speech pathologist should use his or her own judgment and when in doubt, document, document, document! Complete documentation will allow a court to understand why certain decisions were made. It will provide a clear picture of the facts and circumstances of the situation from which to determine whether the speech pathologist acted in accordance with the standard of care under the circumstances. Remember, the test will be what is reasonable, considering the totality of the circumstances. The involvement of the family and the clinician's incorporation of the involvement will be part of that totality.

Speech pathologists may decide that they cannot continue to treat a patient under circumstances that they believe are unsafe. In these situations, speech pathologists do have the option of ending the provider/patient relationship. However, the law does not allow a provider to abandon a patient. If a patient requires continued treatment, the speech pathologist must continue to treat the patient until reasonable arrangements for the assumption of care by another clinician are made. However, practical considerations may make it impossible to change providers. For example, the speech pathologist may practice in a one-clinician hospital. In that case, documentation is even more important to explain the speech pathologist's actions.

Relationship with the Treating Physician

Sometimes the speech pathologist and the treating physician have differing opinions regarding the treatment that a patient should receive. The physician may respond to pressure from the family to provide a certain treatment that the speech pathologist believes is unsafe and inappropriate. What is the standard of care in these situations? Again, it depends on the specific facts involved. It would be impossible to discuss all of the possible scenarios and the standard of care applicable to each one. As with the issues discussed previously, a speech pathologist may follow two important guidelines regarding the speech pathologist's relationship with the physician. These are: (1) ensure that the patient is safe with any treatment provided, and (2) document clearly and completely.

As mentioned previously, safety is key. If a clinician treats a patient in an unsafe manner, a court will likely impose liability, even if the physician requested the treatment. If a speech pathologist, using his or her clinical judgment, determines that a treatment is absolutely unsafe, the speech pathologist may have a responsibility to decline to perform that treatment. A court may not absolve the speech pathologist of liability merely because the physician negligently ordered the treatment. If safety is the first priority, the likelihood of liability may be greatly diminished.

When the speech pathologist's opinion differs from that of the physician, it is essential that the speech pathologist document the circumstances clearly and completely. Include at least the following information in the patient's medical record:

1. Document the presence of conferences with the physician.
2. Clearly document the difference of opinion with the physician and the physician's stated reasons for his or her opinion.
3. Document the speech pathologist's safety concerns regarding the physician's proposed options.
4. Document the speech pathologist's specific recommendations to the physician and reasons for these recommendations.

5. Document the physician's refusal to follow the speech pathologist's recommendations.

Remember, the physician also must meet a standard of care. Clear and complete documentation will help demonstrate whether the clinician has done what is reasonable under the circumstances and whether the physician may have breached the physician's own standard of care.

Relationship with Third-Party-Payers

The age of managed care has ushered in the advent of "prior authorization" for treatment. What is the speech pathologist's duty of care if a payer denies authorization for treatment the speech pathologist feels is medically necessary? Courts have ruled that a health care provider retains the right and the *legal and ethical obligation* to provide appropriate treatment for the patient whether or not the proposed treatment has been approved by the payer.[20] The speech pathologist cannot abdicate his or her obligation to provide appropriate treatment based merely on whether or not the payer will pay for a procedure.

If a payer denies authorization, the clinician should consult with the family. If the family consents to treatment knowing there may be an issue regarding payment, the speech pathologist should continue treatment, assuming, of course, that the treatment is medically necessary.

Recently, courts have ruled that payers can be held liable for harm to a patient caused by negligent utilization review decisions. For example, in *Wickline v. California*,[21] the California state Medicaid program refused to extend a hospital stay for a patient with peripheral vascular disease. The physician discharged the patient without protesting the decision to the payer. Shortly thereafter, the patient's leg became infected and had to be amputated. The court concluded that the physician alone was liable for the harm caused by the patient's early discharge *because he did not contest the decision of the payer* to discharge the patient.[22] However, the court also stated that third-party payers could be held liable for "defects in the design or *implementation* of cost containment mechanisms" that result in the denial of medically necessary services.[23] Although the court did not find the payer negligent in the *Wickline* case, the decision recognizes that negligent utilization review decisions by payers may result in the denial of needed treatment, thereby causing injury to the patient and liability of the payer for negligence.

The courts expanded the concept of payer liability for negligent utilization review decisions in *Wilson v. Blue Cross of Southern California.*[24] In *Wilson*, a boy was admitted to a hospital psychiatric ward for clinical depression and drug dependency. The boy was discharged after a few days because the insurance company declined to approve more than 10 days of hospital care. Shortly after discharge, the boy committed suicide. The court ruled that the insurance company's actions were a "substantial factor" in bringing about the boy's suicide.[25]

These cases show the difficulty of balancing the health care provider's right to treat a patient unencumbered by the payer's treatment decisions and the payer's right to control costs. The lesson here is that a health care provider still may be liable for negligence regardless of the payer's decisions regarding payment. In addition, the payer also may be liable for its own negligent utilization review decisions.

Speech pathologists should consider certain factors when they disagree with a payer's utilization review decision. First, the treating clinician's judgment often receives great deference in a malpractice case, compared to the payer's. Thus, a speech pathologist's actions should not fall below the standard of care regardless of the actions of the payer. Second, the payer's utilization review decisions do not absolve the treating clinician from liability. Thus, acquiescing to the payer's decision may not absolve the clinician from malpractice. Third, the payer's utilization review decisions must be consistent with the same standard of care applicable to the speech pathologist. Thus, a payer's denial of treatment must meet the same clinical standards as the decisions of speech pathologists themselves.

What can speech pathologists do to protect themselves when a payer denies authorization of a treatment that the speech pathologist believes is medically necessary? Several actions are available for speech pathologists that may decrease their liability in these situations.

1. The speech pathologist should provide all relevant information to the payer, whether requested or not.
2. The speech pathologist should verify the exact basis for the utilization review denial.
3. The speech pathologist should articulate to the payer the risks and dangers of failing to provide the requested treatment.
4. The speech pathologist should insist on review of the decision by another speech pathologist.
5. The speech pathologist should inform the patient of the speech pathologist's recommendations, the payer's response, and the risks of not providing treatment.
6. The speech pathologist should request the payer to reconsider the denial, and use any available formal appeals process.
7. The speech pathologist should submit updated patient information to the payer.
8. The speech pathologist should consider expedited court relief.
9. The speech pathologist should resolve all doubts in favor of patient safety.
10. The speech pathologist should remember the "golden rule"—document, document, document.

If speech pathologists take these actions, they should be able to argue that they have done what is reasonable in these situations and have, therefore, met the standard of care.

CONCLUSION

Concern regarding professional negligence is increasing. Speech and language pathologists are at risk for liability, especially in the complex treatment of patients with dysphagia. This chapter attempted to explain in simple terms the basic elements of professional negligence and provide guidelines for minimizing the risks involved. However, it is difficult to discuss all possible factual scenarios because the standard of care depends on the totality of the facts of each situation. Each situation will have its own unique set of facts and circumstances that will influence whether liability will be imposed.

A health care provider has a duty to do what is reasonable under the circumstances. In view of the complexity of the treatments and evaluation tools involved in dysphagia practice, the profession itself may do well to begin addressing liability issues by creating national standards and practice protocols in this area. These standards and protocols may help define the standard of care and give speech and language pathologists guidance in this complex area of clinical practice.

REFERENCES

1. *Agnew v. Parks*, 172 Cal.App.2d 756 (1959).
2. *Brown v. Colm*, 11 Cal.3d 639, 114 Cal.Rptr. 128 (1974). *Bardessono v. Michels*, 3 Cal.3d 780, 91 Cal.Rptr. 760 (1970).
3. *Jamison v. Lindsay*, 108 Cal.App.3d 223, 166 Cal.Rptr. 443 (1980).
4. 36 Cal Jur 3d, Healing Arts and Institutions, Section 156.
5. *Id.*
6. *Id.*
7. *Id.*
8. For example, a neurosurgeon would be held to a higher standard of care than a family practitioner.
9. *Kite v. Campbell*, 142 Cal.App.3d 793, 191 Cal.Rptr. 363 (1983).
10. *Sim v. Weeks*, 7 Cal.App. 28 (1907).
11. *Clemens v. Regents of University of California*, 8 Cal.App.3d 1, 87 Cal.Rptr. 108 (1970).
12. 6 Witkin, 9th ed. Torts, Section 968.
13. *Id.*
14. *Id.*
15. *Id.*
16. *Id.*

17. *Id.*

18. *Bouvia v. Superior Court*, 179 Cal.App.3d 1127, 225 Cal.Rptr. 297 (1986).

19. *Thor v. Superior Court*, 5 Cal.4th 725, 21 Cal.Rptr.2d 357, (1993). This assumes the family member making the decision has the legal competency to make such decisions.

20. *Varol v. Blue Cross & Blue Shield*, 708 F. Supp. 826 (E.D.Mich. 1989).

21. 192 Cal.App.3d 1630, 239 Cal.Rptr. 810 (1986).

22. *Id.*

23. *Id.* (Emphasis added.)

24. 222 Cal.App.3d 660 (1990).

25. *Id.* at 672.

CHAPTER 5

Ethical Considerations in Dysphagia Treatment and Research: Secular and Sacred

Evan G. DeRenzo

Ethical problems that arise while caring for patients with dysphagia are not new, but wide discussions of these problems have been appearing regularly in the literature only for little more than a decade. This literature is focused primarily on the ethical aspects of withholding or withdrawing artificial food and fluids from older adults (Campbell-Taylor & Fisher, 1987; Ciocon, Silverstone, Graver, & Foley, 1988; Volicer, Seltzer, Rheaume, Karner, Glennon, Riley, & Crino, 1989; Ciocon, 1990; Kayser-Jones, 1990; Hodges & Tolle, 1994; Leff, Cheuvront, & Russell, 1994). Additionally, only rare publications examine informed consent regarding the treatment and rehabilitation of dysphagic patients (Krynski, Tymchuk, & Ouslander, 1994), tube feeding from the ethico-legal perspective of least restrictive alternative (Scofield, 1991), and studies of physician attitudes about their perceived obligations to provide or withhold tube feeding (Hodges, Tolle, Stocking, & Cassel, 1994).

As a result of the increasing use of life-extending technologies and the associated increases in costs of care, the President's Commission for the Study of Ethical Problems in Medicine and Biomedical and Behavioral Research examined the is-

The author thanks the following persons for providing critical reviews of this manuscript: David Thomasma, PhD, Loyola University, Chicago, Illinois, and The Rev. Jeanne Brennais, Hospice of Northern Virginia.

Note: The ideas and opinions expressed in this chapter are those of the author only and do not represent any position or policy of the National Institutes of Health, any other Federal agency, or any other institution or organization to which the author is affiliated.

sue of terminating life-extending technologies (President's Commission, 1983). Cases involving termination of treatment, such as those of Clare Conroy and Nancy Cruzan, have produced a flurry of articles (e.g., Annas, 1985a and b; Lo & Dornbrand, 1986), the body of literature addressing ethical concerns in dysphagia is surprisingly small. The reasons for this are open to speculation.

One possibility is that ethical consideration of these issues parallels the introduction of medical technologies, focusing thoughts and discussions narrowly in that direction and away from broader exploration of other sources of moral input. The technical complexities of implementing and managing the many available life-extending technologies may cause the influence of the deeper meanings humans attach to eating and swallowing to go unnoticed. To ensure that these less explicit medical influences that affect our decision-making process are recognized so we can appropriately incorporate them into our moral discussions about dysphagic patients, this chapter seeks to broaden the range of considerations related to the ethical aspects of this condition. Attempts to achieve this goal will be approached from two directions. First, procedural analysis strategies that can be applied to cases as they arise in clinical practice will be presented. Learning how ethical perspectives affect professional recommendations and personal moral preferences will be emphasized. The chapter's second section will explore health care professionals' deeper understandings (i.e., the sacred and secular meanings) involved in decision-making regarding the care of adults and children with dysphagia. This chapter will conclude with recommendations for public policy development and the direction of future research.

PROCEDURAL ETHICS OF DYSPHAGIA: APPLYING ETHICAL ANALYSIS STRATEGIES TO THE TREATMENT AND RESEARCH PARTICIPATION OF ADULTS AND CHILDREN WITH DYSPHAGIA

For clinicians working with dysphagic patients, and the patients' families, friends, and significant others, making ethical judgments is a regular part of clinical care and research participation. Learning systematic ways of analyzing and resolving such questions, however, is not often included in clinical or research training. Using some basic strategies for analyzing ethical issues can help avoid contentious ethical dilemmas and answer the ethical questions that arise in everyday practice. Whether in the clinical care or research setting, clinicians are trained to uphold the basic biomedical principles of beneficence, respect for persons, and justice.

The *principle of beneficence* calls for health care professionals to do or promote the good for the patient or research subject. This principle is the bedrock of all health care ethics, requiring that health care professionals consistently act in the patient's best interest. In so doing, we (health care professionals) work diligently not to breach the oldest biomedical ethical principle, the *principle of nonmalefi-cence*, which requires that we do no harm.

Respect for persons, or what is often referred to as the *principle of autonomy*, requires that we respect individuals as self-determining agents and that we assist persons with making decisions that are consistent with their own values. The *principle of respect* for persons further requires that when an adult's autonomy is impaired or limited (as is often the case with dysphagic patients) or when a minor's autonomy is lacking by definition, we provide the necessary supports and protections to assist such individuals with meeting their presently, or at least previously, held values as much as possible. When an individual's ability to be self-determining is absent and we have no way of knowing what that adult's or child's values are, we act, to the best of our ability, in that adult's or child's best interest, reverting to the dictates of the principle of beneficence.

Often, learning about the patient's values can be made easier by identifying an ethically and legally valid surrogate. The surrogate, when available, or the health care team, if no identifiable surrogate can be located, makes decisions that respect the autonomy of the patient by attempting first to apply a *standard of substituted judgment*. That is, whenever possible, whoever speaks for the patient makes the decisions the patient would have made for him- or herself to the degree those preferences are known.

There are going to be instances, however, when the patient's preferences before the injury and/or disease are unknown or are rendered moot because of his or her present circumstances. For example, in the rehabilitation of persons with traumatic brain injury, frequently the values a patient held before the injury are now irrelevant because of the patient's present and future situations. Or, the patient may not be cognitively aware of what his or her previous wishes were. Therefore, instances will occur when applying a standard of substituted judgment is not considered to be reasonable. At that point, we consider a *standard of best interest*. While considering this standard, we are not neglecting the principle of respect for persons or autonomy, but acting it out under the broader principle of beneficence (Pellegrino & Thomasma, 1988).

The *principle of justice* demands that we act fairly when dealing with our patients and research subjects. That is, we are required to: (1) seek a reasonably equitable balance between benefits and burdens, and (2) create a fair distribution of the goods of health care, and the rest of society's goods, such as clean air and safe streets, among individuals.

Knowing and understanding the central requirements of these basic ethical principles, however, is only the first step in developing strategies for ethical analysis and resolving disagreements that arise in clinical practice, where competing moral claims are part of daily activities. How these principles are applied depends on many factors, including the moral perspectives each health care professional brings to a particular case, the policies and procedures of the institution in which a specific situation occurs, and real or perceived legal constraints.

Case 1: Ethical Considerations

A 76-year-old man who lives at home with his wife has a stroke. This man had executed advance directives making his wife his surrogate decision-maker. He had included in his directives that he does not want to be fed or hydrated through artificial means.

Before the stroke, which has left him unable to communicate or swallow, he was healthy and active. Although his age is a poor prognostic factor, his previous health status is not representative of others his age because of his previous physically active lifestyle. His physicians believe that there is a good chance that he could return to close to normal function during the first several weeks after his stroke. His wife believes that when he documented his preferences not to receive these medical interventions, he had not considered that he might be in a potentially reversible state. His wife wants him to be fed and hydrated through artificial means.

How do you assess this man's previously expressed wishes? Do you believe that inserting a nasogastric or gastrostomy tube would be violating this man's autonomy? Or do you think that regardless of what it appears he wanted, the potential for benefit requires you to override his apparent wishes? Regardless of what his written wishes were, do you believe you must attempt to preserve life? How possible do you think it is that if he is artificially fed and hydrated and returns to baseline function, he will be grateful or inclined to litigate? Regardless of which were to occur, should either possibility influence your prospective decision-making?

Your own values, in large part, will determine how you sort through these questions. Although deeply held, these values and moral perspectives often are not articulated. We often believe that something is the correct thing to do without being completely certain why we feel this way.

Although, as health care professionals, we take care in knowing the scientific justifications for our medical-related recommendations, often we are not as knowledgeable about the source(s) of our own justifications for recommendations that are more value-laden. Furthermore, when we think we are making a recommendation based on objective, scientific, medical grounds, often there are moral values embedded of which we are not even aware.

If, however, we are to act in the best interests of our patients and research subjects, we need to be aware of the values involved in medical recommendations and decisions so that our own biases, and moral and psychological filters do not inadvertently harm our patients and research subjects. One important way to guard against this harm is to analyze our sources of moral knowledge as rigorously as we do our sources of scientific knowledge. Doing so in everyday practice is not as difficult as it might at first seem.

PRINCIPLES OF CLINICAL ETHICS

In clinical ethics, our moral conclusions—consciously or subconsciously—come from only a few major theoretical perspectives within the traditions of Western medicine and philosophy. Becoming more aware of these theories, or world views, allows us to more clearly analyze the moral justifications that underlie the recommendations we make.

Ethical Theories

First, the three traditional ethical theoretical frameworks are consequentialism, deontology, and virtue ethics. Additionally, two newer theoretical frameworks are feminist and communitarian ethics. After learning the basics of these five frameworks (Beauchamp & Childress, 1994), it is easier to understand why, when we are in the midst of ethical debate, we are inclined to balance the ethical principles in one way rather than another. When we become more aware of which ethical perspective(s) we are applying (that is, when we become more self-monitoring about the ethical filters we apply), we are better able to make sound ethical judgments and recommendations. The patient or subject's well-being is enhanced, and the cooperation and function of the health care team is improved.

Consequentialism

Let us first consider one of the most commonly and off-handedly applied theories, consequentialism. A consequentialist perspective postulates that the way to determine whether an action is "right" or "wrong" is by determining whether the consequences of that action will be "good" or "bad." Consequentialism requires that we maximize good and minimize bad outcomes. Consequentialism urges us to produce the greatest good for the greatest number of persons.

We make decisions based on consequentialist analysis every day. For example, think of the nursing home resident with Alzheimer's disease who is beginning to have problems swallowing. This particular resident never stated whether she would want to receive food and hydration artificially, but we know that every time this resident has had to be hospitalized with an intravenous (IV) tube she has become obviously distressed. Her distress has been so great that she has had to be sedated and mittened to prevent her from pulling the IV out. Also, she has a loving husband who, although he admits that he and his wife never discussed these issues explicitly, believes his wife would not want to be kept alive by artificial means in her demented state. He thinks that, although she was a "fighter," she would deem the consequences of the intervention—prolongation of her life in a demented state by artificial means—so harmful to her dignity and psychological well-being that they would outweigh the beneficial consequences of extending her physical life. In this case, our best judgment is that this patient's values before being afflicted with this disease allow us to conclude that she would believe that death may be preferable to life in a demented state sustained by medical intervention.

Consequentialism is an important theory and a useful and practical tool for assessing what ought to be done in many circumstances. But, like most theories, consequentialism has its shortcomings. The primary weakness of consequentialist theory is that it is often difficult or impossible to anticipate what consequences an action may have. Consider a research study in which a new device is being tested for administering food and hydration to critically ill newborns. Although the device has been tested on adults and older children with dysphagia, there can be no guarantee that the device will work when applied to neonates, either on a short- or long-term basis. It is possible that even if no immediate adverse events occur, problems in the infant's development could arise weeks or months later as a direct or indirect result of the experimental device's use. Thus, one must to be cautious when applying a consequentialist analysis, given the difficulties of assessing short- and long-term consequences.

Another drawback of this theoretical framework relates to justice issues and general versus specific consequences. If we believe the consequentialist dictum that we are to maximize the greatest good for the greatest number of persons, what should we do when we are caring for a particular individual? For example, what if a skilled nursing facility has enough staff to monitor dysphagic residents who have nasogastric or gastrostomy tubes, but not enough staff to hand-feed those who require maximal feeding assistance? Does the facility encourage physicians to recommend that residents who might be managed at a lower level of technologic intervention be fed and hydrated through artificial means simply because the consequences for the majority of patients would be safer? To what degree should we tolerate potentially bad consequences for some to maximize potentially good outcomes for many? And, in this particular case, what is a good and what is a bad outcome, for whom, and by whose assessment? Is safety for the greatest number of persons better or worse and from whose perspective when achieving safety means providing nutrition in ways that may constrain personal independence and may compromise individual dignity?

Deontology

The second of the three major ethical theoretical frameworks, deontology, may offer some insights. Deontology bases ethics on meeting one's duties and obligations to individuals. Deontologists believe that some behaviors are morally obligatory, regardless of their consequences. This does not mean that deontologists consider consequences unimportant. Rather, a deontologic perspective accepts that we ought to work toward good consequences whenever possible but that consequences are not the final determinant of right and wrong. Instead, the degree to which one meets one's duties and obligations is, according to a deontologic framework, how we decide whether an action is right or good.

Let us again refer to the 76-year-old man who had a stroke. Remember that this patient had executed advance directives indicating that he did not want to be fed or hydrated through artificial means. His wife, however, wants him to be fed and hydrated through artificial means because his physicians believe his stroke symptoms are reversible and she believes that when her husband documented his preferences he had not anticipated such a possibility.

From a deontologic perspective, what are the duties and obligations of the consulting rehabilitation specialist? The codes of ethics for all health care professionals require that when uncertainty exists, err on the "side of life" and that, when possible, function is to be increased. Additionally, health care professionals must honor the wishes of their patients and clients, to the greatest degree appropriate.

Just from considering this brief scenario, it is clear that determining what one's professional duties and obligations are in a particular case may be as difficult as anticipating consequences. Clarifying these professional duties and obligations can be even more difficult when professionals deeply believe that they should view others as persons before viewing them as patients or research subjects. For example, perhaps one's religious faith teaches that maintaining life, even if doing so limits or overrides personal autonomy, is the greatest good. If one works in an environment where the professionals and the patients or clients all hold the same religious beliefs, no conflicts may arise. But in today's culturally diverse society, the chances are unlikely that personal and professional values will match. Furthermore, professionals involved in any one case may have different perceptions of their duties and obligations. Each medical discipline's codes of ethics are similar, but the nuances to each set of codes are different and can be interpreted differently.

Thus, like consequentialism, deontology helps us to make moral decisions but does not provide us with concrete answers. The last of the three major theoretical frameworks, virtue ethics, also guides us in making good decisions but has its own weaknesses, as well.

Virtue Ethics

Virtue ethics is the oldest of the three Western theoretical frameworks. Dating back to Aristotle, virtue ethics holds that although we should not disregard consequences and meeting our duties and obligations, neither is the final determinant of what is right. Instead, ensuring that your motive is virtuous is fundamentally most important.

Although we often try to consider intuitively another's motive or intent when we are judging his or her behavior, and intent is central to our system of jurisprudence, it is difficult to ever know what really motivates another to behave in a certain way. Much of the field of psychology is devoted to the study of motive and intent, but little of these complex human phenomena are well understood. At times, we even question our ability to understand our own behavior. Determining what motivates another is particularly difficult. Furthermore, philosophers and theologians have been trying to agree on a commonly acceptable list of virtues throughout the centuries, and even now, consensus has yet to be reached.

Considering once again the 76-year-old man who suffered a stroke, for example, if we believe that his wife's request to administer food and fluids through artificial means is motivated by her love for him and her belief that he will recover, we would probably interpret her request as being ethical, even if we disagreed that food and fluids should be administered artificially. But if we thought her request was driven by her fear of being alone, our evaluation of the same behavior might be different, regardless of our own beliefs about what intervention(s) ought to be provided or withheld.

Thus, all three of the most commonly discussed traditional Western ethical theories provide insights but no clear-cut answers. Furthermore, each has fundamental weaknesses; therefore, it may be inadequate to rely on any one of these frameworks as our sole guide to ethical decision-making. This disinclination to rely on any one of these traditional theoretical constructs is strengthened by the advent of two newer perspectives, those of feminist (Tong, 1993; Holmes & Purdy, 1992; Harding, 1991) and communitarian (Cladis, 1992; Loewy, 1991; Emanuel, 1991) ethical theories.

Feminist Ethics

Feminist ethics, in its broadest sense, teaches that, in addition to more traditional ethical considerations, the goodness of an act depends on the specific context in which it occurs. Feminist ethicists state that persons do not make moral decisions in isolation, but rather in relationship to others. A central tenet of feminist ethics, contrary to the assumptions of the three traditional frameworks, is that all persons are interrelated and interdependent, and therefore we make moral decisions in context, not in the abstract.

Feminist ethics may, more precisely, be thought of as a conglomerate of three primary subgroups: liberal, cultural, and radical; each with a different approach to considering gender differences. The liberal view suggests that we ought to focus less on gender differences and treat both genders equally. The cultural view suggests that although gender differences may be as great as have been assumed historically, the problem lies in viewing these differences pejoratively, rather than as reason for celebration. The radical perspective, like the cultural perspective, focuses on the differences between the sexes, but focuses on the darker side of these gender differences, largely by focusing on power and oppression.

In the case of the 76-year-old patient who had a stroke, a feminist perspective suggests that we need to examine closely the contextual aspects of the case. Do members of the health care team disagree with each other about the potential for this man's impairments to be reversed? And if so, who is in disagreement? Is the physician recommending aggressive intervention the powerful attending physician, whose religious background encourages him to sustain life at all cost, whereas those suggesting that reversibility is not so likely are the residents or nurses? Regardless of the particular theoretical emphasis one chooses, a feminist ethics approach teaches us that contextual factors, such as the life experiences of the parties involved, provide important information and must be considered if we are to arrive at ethically justifiable decisions.

Communitarianism

The final theoretical perspective is communitarianism. Communitarianism teaches that, in addition to the considerations raised by the previously mentioned four theories, the goodness of an act depends, also, on its broader social context. That is, considerations of social context, social history, and the customs and moral norms of specific communities are morally relevant factors in the ethical analysis of a particular case. For the 76-year-old man who had a stroke, communitarian ethics require that we consider the values about artificially administered food and fluids held by this patient's wife and other family members, as well as the beliefs and norms about life-extending technologies held by the religious and ethnic groups of both the patient and his wife.

This concludes the brief overview of the basic ethical principles and the main theoretical perspectives, or world views, that influence the judgments of persons and professionals and shapes their recommendations about how best to care for children and adults with dysphagic disorders. Professionals must be aware that these judgments and recommendations often are value-laden. But knowing the basic ethical principles of beneficence, respect for persons, and justice is only the first step in developing strategies for ethical analysis. Being able to identify and separate the components of fundamental theories during an ethical discussion is the second step. The third, and final, step is determining what information and processes are needed to appropriately address the many ethical issues that arise during the care or study of dysphagic patients (Haas & Malouf, 1989; Drane, 1988; Geary, 1988).

CREATING ETHICAL PROCEDURES

This third and final step starts at the fact-finding stage. When an ethical question arises, sufficient depth and scope of information and perceptions about the medical, psychological, social, and contextual factors should be gathered. These data are necessary to be able to consider the major issues related to the case. This includes the history of the case, including legal and institutional history. Document who thinks which principles are in conflict and why they think so. That is, listen to as many of the people involved as possible. Have them express what values they believe are at stake. Listen closely to understand in which theoretical framework each person is grounding her or his perspective on the case.

Become sensitive to the pressure points in the system or case while documenting and organizing these facts, perceptions, and opinions. That is, notice who speaks more freely when various persons are or are not present. Keep attuned to how conversations occur when persons of differing power relate to each other. Be sensitive to nonverbal language. Be alert to subtle misunderstandings stemming from gender or cultural differences. Note who is driving the process. Who is blocking a consensus? Why are they not able or willing to join those in the mainstream? Around which persons and options is a consensus growing? Do those in agreement truly agree with each other or are they just tired or fearful?

Once a critical mass of information has been gathered and discussions have occurred, identify the full range of ethically acceptable and clinically probable solutions. Work collaboratively to evaluate the benefits and limitations of each option. Then make certain that the necessary psychological and institutional supports for implementing the best decision are provided.

Cases in which swallowing is impaired regularly raise many difficult moral questions. Each person involved in a case will bring to it notions, often unarticulated, of how best to care for persons who cannot feed themselves, how important eating and swallowing are to the quality of one's life, how vigorously sustaining that life should be pursued and what the boundary is between seeking the good life and smoothing the way toward a good death. And, like the rapid changes that can occur in patients and research subjects clinically, how we weigh a particular moral judgment or recommendation will be related to the changing mix of clinical circumstances. That is why it is wise for all clinicians to learn the basics of ethical analysis and develop a decision-making process (akin to the decision-analysis strategies commonly applied during the diagnostic process) to help deal with the difficult moral issues that arise while studying dysphagia and treating dysphagic patients.

PHILOSOPHIC MEANINGS RELATED TO DYSPHAGIA: SACRED AND SECULAR VALUES

No matter how well one can analyze and resolve ethical dilemmas that arise while caring for adults and children with dysphagia, ethical decisions often are difficult and emotionally painful. This seems true especially when these decisions involve initiating, withholding, or withdrawing life-extending technologies.

Decisions to initiate, withhold, or withdraw artificially administered foods and fluids seem more difficult to make, emotionally, than decisions about other life-extending technologies. Even though guidelines for the termination of these interventions have been published (The Hastings Center, 1987), and the Supreme Court decision in the Nancy Cruzan case identifies artificially administered nutrition and hydration as a medical intervention like any other, withholding or withdrawing these technologies seems to be more heart-wrenching than withholding or withdrawing other life-extending technologies. Why might this be?

Although this should be empirically verified, it seems that the deeper meanings associated with the acts of eating and swallowing are the source of the profound emotional and psychological discomforts at the prospect of withholding or withdrawing artificially administered nutrition and hydration. Our deeply held and often subconscious beliefs related to feeding, swallowing, and communicating may make our decisions to initiate, withhold, or withdraw artificially administered food and hydration seem even more difficult than those regarding other life-extending technologies, such as ventilatory support or administration of antibiotics.

Infectious agents and lack of air kill as surely as lack of food and water. But neither air nor infections are consciously exchanged as part of our daily activities. Neither are visible to the human eye. Air is taken for granted until it becomes so polluted that we must act to restore its suitability. The viruses and bacteria that produce infections are ubiquitous and ignored until they produce disease requiring aggressive intervention. Both air and infectious agents enter our bodies unseen and unnoticed, and we do not think about them during our daily lives.

Provision of food and fluids is qualitatively different. Solid and liquid nourishments are visible aspects of our environment, and they are necessities of life we give to each other. Food and fluids visibly enter our bodies through our mouths, which we use to communicate with one another. Social customs are involved in eating and drinking in every social group from preliterate to highly technologic societies. Ritualistic eating and drinking are part of our most common daily activities and our most important secular and religious practices. Food customs and religious dietary laws delineate social relationships by establishing and maintaining boundaries between and among social groups, and providing individuals within groups with a sense of social identity.

Considering the many ways in which eating and swallowing are integral to how we relate to each other, what deeper meanings do professionals, family members, and friends bring to the bedside of adults and children with dysphagia? Why are decisions involved with the technologic treatment of dysphagic patients qualitatively different, emotionally, from those involving the technologic treatment of other kinds of equally grave disorders and conditions? When acting as a professional and making recommendations or acting as a family member or friend and expressing preferences for care of patients with dysphagic disorders, what lies beneath our words and conscious thoughts? What meanings and symbols about eating and swallowing shape our biases and our moral filters? The remainder of this section will discuss just a fraction of what these deeply ingrained meanings may be.

SYMBOLISM OF EATING AND DRINKING AMONG SOCIETIES

Although there are no universal food customs or dietary laws, every society, from preliterate to technologic, develops eating and drinking customs and attaches symbolic value to certain foods and ways of consuming specific nutrients. These customs dictate what may and may not be consumed, at what times, and in what places. Most often, these customs have little to do with nutritive factors but are, instead, designed to delineate and solidify social relationships.

Religious Behaviors and Eating

Religious and secular ceremonies are replete with ritualistic eating and drinking behaviors symbolizing life and merriment. The gaiety of the bacchanal continues to symbolize life and vitality to this day. The provision of food and drink, whether or not actual feasting occurs, is characteristic of most rites of passage. Nowhere is this more evident than at weddings. Wedding ceremonies around the world include ritualistic eating and drinking.

Religious food rituals, designed to separate social groups, continue today in every religious group. This intensity of members bonding to each other and separating from those who do not have the same beliefs through religious customs involving food and drink can be seen in Christianity, in Judaism, and among U.S. African Americans who have become members of the Nation of Islam. Meals serve to equalize social status rather than to stratify. In religions originating in India, primarily Hinduism but also Jainism and Sikhism, the relationships between ritualistic eating and social stratification are most clearly observed. Food customs help define caste ranking.

Secular Behaviors and Rituals

Changing focus from the explicitly religious to the deeper meanings about eating that merge sacred and secular values, sharing food symbolizes trust. Often, saying, "We eat together" is saying, "We trust each other, even if we are not members of the same tribe or kin." This is as true for the Nyakyusa of Tanzania as for teenagers in a U.S. high school cafeteria. The meanings we attach to eating, drinking, and swallowing are connected to our most cherished activities and remind us of the intangibles of human existence—trust, dependence, social worth, and love—and, therefore, become integral to how we see ourselves as individuals and in relation to others.

Perhaps the most pervasive, eternal, and primitive image of feeding and swallowing is that of a mother nursing her infant. Sucking and swallowing are universally understood to be psychologically soothing behaviors. When an infant cries, the seemingly evolutionarily programmed response is to bring that infant to the mother's breast to feed. We all recognize that process as not only nutritive for the infant, but psychologically calming for both mother and child. Later in their lives, after children have been weaned, some will suck their thumb as a self-soothing behavior reminiscent of suckling their mother's breast. This search for self-soothing eating and swallowing substitutes can continue throughout one's life. Food or fluids are regularly used for psychological relief.

As the Japanese tea ceremony and the British custom of high tea are examples of small-scale images that serve as powerful metaphors for our social interactions and personal development, the social miseries of famine, poverty, and its related hunger are large-scale images that also affect us. For anyone who has ever been hungry, the prospect of thinking of a loved one dying from hunger can be particularly frightening and repugnant. Nations have migrated to avoid hunger and famine. The images we carry of seeing children with bellies swollen from malnutrition are strong disincentives to depriving others of food and water, even when medical interventions that appear to minimize the sensations of hunger and thirst are practiced (McCann, Hall, & Groth-Juncker, 1994).

For so many of us throughout history and around the world, exchange of food and drink was and is at the core of our most important human activities—from foods sacrificed to the gods, and goats and oxen given as gifts to the tribe of the newly betrothed, to fancy sweet breads given to our relatives and friends at holidays, and drinking champagne to celebrate our most important successes. These, and many more, are the experiences we as professionals, patients, and family members bring to our decision-making about how to care for adults and children with diseases that impair, interrupt, or preclude normal eating, swallowing, and communicating. And, this emotional, psychological, and spiritual framework may, in large part, make decision-making regarding dysphagic patients and research subjects so difficult.

CONCLUSION: RECOMMENDATIONS FOR PUBLIC POLICY AND FUTURE RESEARCH

How, then, are we supposed to apply the many meanings and beliefs we have about eating and swallowing to everyday practice of the clinical care and research participation of adults and children with dysphagic disorders? And do we improve the care of dysphagic patients in ways that also advance the well-being of the society at large?

One way is to create more opportunities to explore our tacit and explicit beliefs about ethical aspects of care for these patients and how these beliefs influence our judgments and recommendations. At the institutional level, this exploration can take the form of expanded discussions on rounds, ethics colloquia and seminars, and ethics columns in internal publications.

At the local government level, state departments of health can establish statewide and regional annual meetings to discuss these complex medical and socially important issues. Such meetings might best be organized to bring professionals who care for persons with dysphagia and similar and/or related disorders together with members of and advocates for specialized patient groups.

In addition, if these meetings occurred across a sufficiently broad cross section of the national population, they could serve as data collection points; large data sets could aid with determining where consensus does and does not exist, and where efforts for public education might be most effectively and efficiently focused. Data analysis could be centralized, for example at the National Institutes of Health, by a federal ethics advisory board, or through a federal grant to a university.

Research in various areas might provide important insights into ethical concerns related to persons with dysphagia. For example, Scofield (1991), in his article on artificial feeding and least restrictive alternative, suggested that decisions to initiate, withhold, or withdraw food and fluids administered through artificial means may not be based on adequate clinical evaluation. Data investigating why and how decisions relating to the care of dysphagic patients are made need to be collected. What variables, obvious and hidden, are involved when such decisions are being made? What are the barriers to making optimal decisions in these cases? What institutional, educational, and psychological supports could be used or created to maximize optimal medico-ethical decision-making for these patients? These questions are amenable to empirical investigation.

Dysphagic patients and the professionals who treat these patients could benefit from research about outcomes. What benefits and burdens do the various interventions attempted in the care of dysphagic patients place on these patients and their caregivers? Given different outcomes, both physical and psychosocial, can we consistently optimize treatment decisions regarding patient parameters such as disease severity, number of other concomitant medical problems, functional status before development of dysphagic disorders, or etiology factors? Which interventions leave the least psychological, spiritual, and fiscal harms after dysphagic patients die? These questions also await research attention.

The medical management of patients with dysphagia is complex and raises many thorny ethical questions. We are forced to examine our beliefs about the benefits and limitations of modern technologic advances, our hopes for life, and our fears about death. Often, it is easier, emotionally, for patients, patients' families, and health care providers not to seek answers to the difficult questions that arise but, rather, seek "quick" fixes through technologic means. We must avoid this and, instead, approach the ethical analyses involved in decision-making regarding these patients with the same rigor that we apply to our scientific analyses. In so doing, we will be seeking the highest ethical standards of conduct in the clinical care and research participation of adults and children with dysphagia.

REFERENCES

Annas, G.J. (1985a). Fashion and freedom: When artificial feeding should be withdrawn. *American Journal of Public Health, 75* (6), 685–688.

Annas, G.J. (1985b). When procedures limit rights: From Quinlan to Conroy. *The Hastings Center Report, 15* (2), 24–26.

Beauchamp T.L., & Childress, J.F. (1994). *Principles of biomedical ethics.* New York: Oxford University Press.

Campbell-Taylor, I., & Fisher, R.H. (1987). The clinical case against tube feeding in palliative care of the elderly. *Journal of the Geriatrics Society, 35,* 1100–1104.

Ciocon, J.O. (1990). Indications for tube feeding in elderly patients. *Dysphagia, 5,* 1–5.

Ciocon, J.O., Silverstone, F.A., Graver, L.M., & Foley, C.J. (1988). Tube feeding in elderly patients: Indications, benefits, and complications. *Archives of Internal Medicine, 148,* 429–433.

Cladis, M.S. (1992). *A communitarian defense of liberalism: Emile Durkeim and contemporary social theory.* Stanford, CA: Stanford University Press.

Emanuel, E.J. (1991). *The ends of human life: Medical ethics in a liberal polity.* Cambridge, MA: Harvard University Press.

Drane, J.F. (1988). "Ethical workup" guides clinical decision making. *Health Progress, December,* 64–67.

Geary, M. (1988). Guidelines for ethical decision making. *Oncology Nursing Forum, 15,* 487.

Guerber, H.A. (1993). *The myths of Greece and Rome.* New York: Dover Publications.

Haas, L.J., & Malouf, J.L. (1989). *Keeping up the good work: A practitioner's guide to mental health ethics.* Sarasota, FL: Professional Resource Exchange, Inc.

Harding, S. (1991). *Whose science? Whose knowledge?: Thinking from women's lives.* Ithaca, NY: Cornell University Press.

The Hastings Center. (1987). *Guidelines on the termination of life-sustaining treatment and the care of the dying.* Bloomington, IN: Indiana University Press.

Hodges, M.O., & Tolle, S.W. (1994). Tube-feeding decisions in the elderly. In G.A. Sachs, & C.K. Cassel (Eds.), *Clinics in geriatric medicine, 10* (3), 475–488.

Hodges, M.O., Tolle, S.W., Stocking, C., & Cassel, C.K. (1994). Tube feeding: Internists' attitudes regarding ethical obligations. *Archives of Internal Medicine, 154,* 1013–1020.

Holmes, H.B., & Purdy, L.M. (1992). *Feminist perspectives in medical ethics.* Bloomington, IN: Indiana University Press.

Kayser-Jones, J. (1990). The use of nasogastric feeding tubes in nursing homes: Patient, family and health care provider perspectives. *The Gerontologist, 30* (4), 469–479.

Krynski, M.D., Tymchuk, A.J., & Ouslander, J.G. (1994). How informed can consent be? New light on comprehension among elderly people making decisions about enteral tube feeding. *The Gerontologist, 34* (1), 36–43.

Leff, B., Cheuvront, N., & Russell, W. (1994). Discontinuing feeding tubes in a community nursing home. *The Gerontologist, 34* (1), 130–133.

Lo, B., and Dornbrand, L. (1986). The case of Claire Conroy: Will administrative review safeguard incompetent patients? *Annals of Internal Medicine, 104,* 869–873.

Loewy, E.H. (1991). *Suffering and the beneficent community: Beyond libertarianism.* Albany, NY: State University of New York Press.

McCann, R.M., Hall, W.S., & Groth-Juncker, A. (1994). Comfort care for terminally ill patients: The appropriate use of nutrition and hydration. *Journal of the American Medical Association, 272* (16), 1263–1266.

Pellegrino, E.D., & Thomasma, D.C. (1988). *For the patient's good: The restoration of beneficence in health care.* New York: Oxford University Press.

President's Commission for the Study of Ethical Problems in Medicine and Biomedical and Behavioral Research. (1983). *Deciding to forego life-sustaining treatment: A report on the ethical, medical and legal issues in treatment decisions.* Washington, DC: U.S. Government Printing Office.

Scofield, G.R. (1991). Artificial feeding: The least restrictive alternative? *The Journal of the Geriatric Society, 39* (12), 1217–1220.

Tong, R. (1993). *Feminine and feminist ethics.* Belmont, CA: Wadsworth Publishing Co.

Volicer, L., Seltzer, B., Rheaume, Y., Karner, J., Glennon, M., Riley, M.E., & Crino, P. (1989). Eating difficulties in patients with probable dementia of the Alzheimer type. *Journal of Geriatric Psychiatry and Neurology, 2* (4), 188–195.

CHAPTER 6

The Effects of Medications on Swallowing

Madeline Feinberg

Medications can play a multifactorial role in the pathogenesis, treatment, and prevention of swallowing disorders. Familiarity with the mechanism of a drug's action and the pathophysiology of the swallowing disorder (if known) can help the clinician identify drugs that may contribute, directly or indirectly, to the swallowing disorder. Suboptimal drug therapy in certain neuromuscular disorders, for example Parkinson's Disease (PD), may predispose the patient to oropharyngeal swallowing dysfunction. In other cases, medications used to treat one medical problem may exacerbate another problem; for example, the use of nitrates to treat coronary artery disease could worsen reflux disease by contributing to lower esophageal sphincter incompetence. Medications also can be the direct cause of the swallowing disorder as seen in pill-induced esophagitis. Medication side effects, notably dry mouth, pharyngeal ulceration, or tardive dyskinesia, may cause or worsen dysphagia. Side effects can be subtle, too, such as anorexia or drug-induced confusion. When this occurs, the patient's rehabilitation or routine care can be significantly compromised.

OROPHARYNGEAL DYSPHAGIA (TRANSFER DYSPHAGIA)

Functionally, the act of swallowing is considered to have three phases: oral, pharyngeal, and esophageal (Richter, 1993). The oral phase consists of the oral preparatory and oral voluntary components, where the food is masticated, transported over the tongue surface, and prepared for swallowing. The pharynx, upper esophageal sphincter, and upper one-third of the esophagus are composed of skeletal muscle. The oropharyngeal phase of swallowing is controlled both voluntarily and involuntarily (Diamant, 1993). The frontal cortex, swallowing center in the brainstem, and sensory feedback mechanisms from the oropharyngeal area function in a coordinated pattern during the swallowing sequence (Diamant, 1993).

The voluntary component of swallowing (oral preparation and oral transport) may be jeopardized by drugs that interfere with cognition or alertness. Confused or sedated patients may have difficulty initiating a swallow. Indeed, patients presenting while confused or sedated can be difficult to assess and treat. In general, elderly patients are most at risk for drug-induced confusion, particularly if a cognitive impairment pre-exists. All medications that act on the central nervous system, most notably the anticholinergics, psychotropics, analgesics, and antiepileptics, have the potential to cause confusion (Sunderland, Tariot, Cohen, Weingartner, Mueller, & Murphy, 1987; Kurlan & Como, 1988; Feinberg, 1993). Drugs most often associated with cognitive impairment are presented in Table 6–1. Many of these medications also cause sedation as well. The risk of adverse reactions associated with cognitive impairment increases with the number of drugs taken (Larson, Kukull, Buchner, & Reifler, 1987). Therefore, every effort should be made to reduce or eliminate medications that can alter mental status, especially when the benefit of the medication is unclear. Drugs likely to cause confusion should be identified before treating patients with dysphagia.

Either structural lesions or neuromuscular disorders cause abnormalities of the pharynx and upper esophageal sphincter (UES). The majority of these neuromuscular disorders are progressive and untreatable (Clouse, 1993). However, for some disorders, drug therapy can be optimized to improve symptoms (Table 6–2).

Approximately 40% of patients with PD present with significant dysphagia, secondary to direct involvement of the oropharyngeal muscles (Koller, Silver, & Lieberman, 1994). Many patients with PD have swallowing dysfunction but remain asymptomatic (Koller et al., 1994). Whereas some patients experience improved swallowing either symptomatically or objectively after levodopa administration, others do not (Bushman, Dobmeyer, Leeker, & Permutter, 1989). A patient with PD should be evaluated for swallowing dysfunction when his or her PD-related symptoms are reasonably well controlled by the medication, that is, when the patient is "on." Appointments for swallowing evaluation should be determined by the patient's medication schedule. The time and dose of the most recent medication should be noted on the evaluation workup for consistent follow-up. In general, patients with PD should be instructed to eat when they are "on," whenever possible (Koller et al., 1994).

Skeletal muscle dysfunction causing dysphagia can be due to hyperthyroidism or hypothyroidism (Cohen, 1979). Administering antithyroid drugs such as propylthiouracil or methimazole (Tapazole) is one of several treatment options available for hyperthyroidism. When antithyroid medications are prescribed, monthly or bimonthly monitoring is required to reassess dosage (Haynes, 1990). Thyroid replacement therapy such as administering Synthroid or thyroid hormone is used to correct hypothyroidism. Once the dosage is stabilized, adult patients usually are monitored annually. A case of dysphagia caused by hypothyroidism

Table 6–1 Drugs Associated with Mental Status Changes, Confusion, and/or Sedation

Drug Class	Selected Examples
Alcohol	Beer, wine, whiskey, vitamin tonics (check alcohol content)
Antianxiety drugs	benzodiazepines (Valium, Xanax, Ativan, Tranxene)
	hydroxyzine (Atarax)*
Anticholinergic drugs	benztropine (Cogentin)*
	biperiden (Akineton)*
	diphenhydramine (Benadryl)*
	procyclidine (Kemadrin)*
	trihexyphenidyl (Artane)*
Antiepileptic drugs	carbamazepine (Tegretol)
	clonazepam (Klonopin)
	phenytoin (Dilantin)
	phenobarbital
Antidepressants	amitriptyline (Elavil)*
	desipramine (Norpramin)*
	doxepin (Sinequan)*
	fluoxetine (Prozac)
	imipramine (Tofranil)*
	nefazodone (Serzone)
	nortriptyline (Pamelor)*
	paroxetine (Paxil)
	sertraline (Zoloft)
	venlafaxine (Effexor)
Antiemetics	meclizine (Antivert)*+
	metoclopramide (Reglan)
	prochlorperazine (Compazine)*
	promethazine (Phenergan)*
Antihistamines	chlorpheniramine (Chlor-Trimeton)*+
	cyproheptadine (Periactin)*
	diphenhydramine (Benadryl)*+
	hydroxyzine (Atarax)*
Antihypertensives	beta blockers (propranolol)
	clonidine (Catapres)
	diuretics (hydrochlorothiazide)
	hydralazine (Apresoline)
	methyldopa (Aldomet)
	propranolol (Inderal)
	reserpine

continues

Table 6–1 continued

Drug Class	Selected Examples
Antiparkinson drugs	amantadine (Symmetrel)
	bromocriptine (Parlodel)
	pergolide (Permax)
	selegiline (Eldepryl)
Antipsychotics	chlorpromazine (Thorazine)*
	clozapine (Clozaril)*
	fluphenazine (Prolixin)*
	haloperidol (Haldol)*
	thioridazine (Mellaril)*
Antitussives	codeine (Robitussin AC)
	Hydromorphone (Dilaudid cough syrup)
Cardiac drugs	digoxin (Lanoxin)
	disopyramide (Norpace)
	procainamide (Procan)
	quinidine (Quinidex)
Decongestants	ephedrine+
	phenylpropanolamine (PPA)+
	pseudoephedrine+ (Sudafed)+
Histamine-2	cimetidine (Tagamet)+
antagonists	ranitidine (Zantac)+
Hypnotics	barbiturates
	benzodiazepines (Dalmane, Doral, ProSom)
	chloral hydrate (Noctec)
	diphenhydramine (Sominex)+
Muscle relaxants	cyclobenzaprine (Flexeril)
	orphenadrine (Norflex)
Narcotic analgesics	codeine (Tylenol #3)
	fentanyl (Duragesic)
	meperidine (Demerol)
	morphine
	pentazocine (Talwin)
	propoxyphene (Darvon)
Nonsteroidal anti-	ibuprofen (Motrin)+
inflammatory drugs	indomethacin (Indocin)
(NSAIDs)	naproxen (Naprosyn)+
	piroxicam (Feldene)
Steroids	dexamethasone (Deltasone)
	prednisone

Note: This list is not complete. (Check with pharmacist for specific medications)
* anticholinergic effects
+ available over the counter (without prescription)

Table 6–2 Selected Diseases/Problems That May Cause Oropharyngeal Dysphagia

Problem	Possible Solution
Parkinson's disease	Optimize dopaminergic therapy; counsel patient to eat when "on."
Hyper/hypothyroidism	Normalize thyroid function.
Steroid myopathy	Reassess steroid therapy. Can patient tolerate dose taper?
Alcoholic myopathy	Identify alcohol abuse; refer for treatment.
Diabetic neuropathy	Achieve desired blood glucose goals; consider referral for diabetes education.
Inflammatory myopathies	Corticosteroid therapy may improve muscle function in dermatomyositis and polymyositis.
Myasthenia gravis	Assess symptom control. Is patient able to titrate dose to response?

with myxedema resolved after a few months of thyroid replacement (Wright & Penner, 1981).

High-dose steroids, when used for long duration, cause skeletal muscle wasting which can manifest as pharyngeal dysphagia (Haynes, 1990). Unfortunately, patients receiving steroids may not be able to tolerate a reduction in dosage, but this should be confirmed by the physician and not assumed by the clinician treating the patient's dysphagia.

Alcoholic myopathy also has been reported to cause pharyngeal dysphagia, probably because of the direct toxic effect of alcohol on the muscle of the pharynx. In previously reported cases, symptoms disappeared after 4 months of significantly reduced alcohol intake (Weber, Nashel, & Mellow, 1981).

Myasthenia gravis, a disease caused by a defect in neurotransmission at the skeletal muscle motor endplate, results in weakness and fatigability, which can impair swallowing. Myasthenia gravis is treated with agents that delay the breakdown of acetylcholine in the synapse, thereby prolonging its action. Pyridostigmine (Mestinon) and ambenonium (Mytelase) are used for chronic treatment. Because this disease can worsen and remit unpredictably, physicians can teach their patients to modify the frequency and size of their dose of medication based on their symptoms (Taylor, 1990).

Diabetic neuropathy, which causes dysphagia-related symptoms, unlike the abnormalities previously mentioned, cannot be corrected by a pharmacologic intervention. However, recent studies suggest that development or progression of the neuropathy can be slowed by improving blood glucose control (The Diabetes Control and Complications Trial Research Group, 1993).

ESOPHAGEAL DYSPHAGIA

The esophageal body (EB) and the lower esophageal sphincter (LES) consist of smooth muscle. Cholinergic neurons innervate both the EB and LES as excitatory neurons. Nonadrenergic noncholinergic neurons (neurotransmitter unknown) innervate the EB and play an inhibitory role. The adrenergic nervous system modulates contraction, amplitude, velocity, and LES tone. Specifically, in the gastrointestinal tract, beta-adrenergic effects appear to inhibit cholinergic transmission, whereas the alpha-adrenergic effect increases cholinergic transmission.

Achalasia

Dysphagia associated with solid foods is almost always reported by patients with achalasia. Achalasia is associated with elevated LES pressure, incomplete LES relaxation, and lack of coordinated contractions throughout the esophagus (Clouse, 1993). Drugs that act on the smooth muscle, nerves, or both may worsen or relieve symptoms depending on the drugs' mechanisms of action (Table 6–3 and 6–4). Treatment is directed at relaxing the LES, preferably using pneumatic polyethylene balloon dilation; however in some patients drugs may be a better option than dilation (Cohen, 1992).

Table 6–3 Drugs That Increase Lower Esophageal Pressure (May Worsen Symptoms of Achalasia)

Drug Class	Examples	Pharmacologic Effect
Antacids	Maalox, Tums	Produces pH-dependent increase in LES pressure (Higgs, Smyth, & Castell, 1974)
Alpha adrenergic agonists	ergonovine	Direct smooth muscle stimulant
Beta adrenergic antagonists	propranolol	Indirectly stimulates acetylcholine release
Cholinergic agonists	bethanechol	Mimics action of acetylcholine
Prokinetic agents	cisapride metoclopramide domperidone	Promotes acetylcholine release

Table 6–4 Drugs That Decrease Lower Esophageal Pressure

Drug Class	Example
Alcohol	ethanol
Alpha adrenergic antagonists	reserpine
Anticholinergic agents	(see Table 6–1)
Barbiturates	phenobarbital
Benzodiazepines	diazepam
Beta adrenergic agonists	terbutaline
Caffeine	
Calcium channel blockers	nifedipine, verapamil, diltiazem
Cigarette smoking	
Dopaminergic drugs	Sinemet, bromocriptine, pergolide
Meperidine	Demerol
Methylxanthines	theophylline, aminophylline
Nitrates	isosorbide dinitrate, nitroglycerin
Progesterone	(high during pregnancy)

The calcium-channel blockers, nitrates, methylxanthines, and beta agonists have been reported to relieve symptoms of achalasia and improve swallowing function. Overall early studies have been disappointing (Castell, 1975). Case reports and uncontrolled studies have documented symptomatic improvement of achalasia with nifedipine (Bortolotti & Labo, 1981; Berger & McCallum, 1982; Traube, Hongo, Magyar, & McCallum, 1984; Thomas, Lebow, Gubler, & Bryant, 1984). However, two blinded crossover studies showed that despite reduction of LES pressure, neither nifedipine nor verapamil produced clinically significant differences in overall symptomatology (Triadafilopoulos, Aaronson, Sackel, & Burakoff, 1991). In one single blinded crossover study, sublingual isosorbide dinitrate was more effective than nifedipine in relieving symptoms (Gelfond, Rozen, & Gilat, 1982). In a three-way open-design crossover study of terbutaline, nitroglycerin, and aminophylline, all drugs decreased LES pressure, but only terbutaline and nitroglycerin significantly improved esophageal emptying in some, but not all, of the subjects (Wong, Maydonovitch, Gargia, Johnson, & Castell, 1987).

Spastic Disorders

A common etiology of noncardiac chest pain is diffuse esophageal spasms, although the incidence may be overestimated (Nostrant, Sams, & Huber, 1986). These are characterized by abnormal nonperistaltic contractions, abnormal contraction wave amplitude and duration, or sporadic, intense contractions (Richter, 1993). Patients may present with symptoms of dysphagia. Interestingly, it has been suggested to use bethanechol, a cholinergic agent, to stimulate the esophagus to aid with identifying the origin of the chest pain (Murad, 1990).

The majority of patients with spastic disorders have normal LES pressure and relaxation despite abnormal esophageal contractions (Cohen, 1979). Because nitrates relax almost all smooth muscle and have been shown to reduce the spontaneous motility of the esophagus in vitro and in vivo, their efficacy in "angina" due to esophageal spasm may be explained (Murad, 1990). "Nutcracker esophagus," which is an increase in distal esophageal contraction amplitude with chest pain, was not improved by nifedipine despite a significant decrease in contraction amplitude (Richter, Dalton, Bradley, & Castell, 1987).

Alcohol exerts opposing effects on esophageal motility depending on whether alcohol intake is acute or chronic. Alcoholics in withdrawal experience abnormally high esophageal contraction amplitude, whereas acute intoxication produces diminished esophageal contraction amplitude (Keshavarzian, Polepalle, Iber, & Durkin, 1990). Abnormal findings in chronic alcoholics have been shown to be reversible after 1 month of sobriety (Keshavarzian, Iber, & Ferguson, 1987).

Gastroesophageal Reflux Disease

Dysphagia is a primary symptom of gastroesophageal reflux disease (GERD) and occurs in about 30% of patients with reflux disease (Kahrilas & Hogan, 1993). The LES functions as a barrier to the reflux of gastric contents. In many, but not all, patients with mild to moderate GERD, LES resting pressure is diminished. Inappropriate relaxation of the LES may be a more common finding in GERD. Factors other than those related to LES competence are important in the pathogenesis of GERD. Inability to clear refluxed acid from the esophagus contributes to GERD. Normally, when acid refluxes into the esophagus, it is cleared by esophageal peristalsis and by saliva, which contains a high amount of bicarbonate (Kahrilas & Hogan, 1993). Saliva substitutes do not contain bicarbonate and do not replace normal saliva function in esophageal acid clearance (Helm, Dodds, Pelc, Palmer, Hogan, & Teeter, 1984). Alcohol, when taken before lying down, has been shown to impair esophageal acid clearance (Vitale, Cheadle, Patel, Sadek, Michel, & Cuschieri, 1987).

Esophageal dysphagia in patients with GERD may be due to the progressive development of strictures (Schatzki rings) in severe GERD (Marshall, Kretschmar, & Diaz-Arias, 1990), but dysphagia is often present without evidence of strictures.

Treatment of GERD is directed at eliminating irritating foods or drugs that lower LES pressure and uses antireflux therapy. Antireflux therapies include antacids, histamine-2 receptor antagonists, proton pump inhibitors, and prokinetic drugs. Antacids neutralize esophageal acid and increase LES pressure. Histamine-2 receptor antagonists (Zantac, Pepsid, Axid, Tagamet) and the proton pump inhibitors omeprazole (Prilosec) and lansoprazole block acid formation, thereby decreasing gastric acidity and reducing the digestive action of pepsin. Proton pump inhibitors are considered to be more effective than the histamine-2 receptor antagonists (H_2RAs) in more severe cases of GERD. Of note, many of the H_2RAs recently have been approved to be distributed "over the counter" in the United States to treat heartburn, a primary symptom of mild GERD. The prokinetic drug cisapride (Propulsid) has been demonstrated to relieve symptoms and promote healing in mild GERD (Klinkenberg-Knol, Festen, & Meuwissen, 1995).

A large number of medications can decrease saliva production, primarily through an anticholinergic mechanism. These are highlighted in Table 6–1. Many other classes of medications, such as decongestants, beta blockers, benzodiazepines, and narcotic analgesics, to name a few, also cause dry mouth via different mechanisms. Medications that inhibit saliva production have been shown to reduce clearance of acid from the esophagus and increase the duration of time that the pH within the esophagus is less than 4.0 compared to normals (Korsten, Rosman, Fishbein, Shlein, Goldberg, & Biener, 1991).

ODYNOPHAGIA

Pain on swallowing is usually the result of an esophageal injury, and often can be caused by a tablet or capsule that lodges or adheres to the mucosal wall of the esophagus (Richter, 1993). Pill-induced esophagitis most often has been reported with tetracycline, doxycycline, minocycline, quinidine, and sustained release potassium chloride (Bott, Prakash, & McCallum, 1987), although a host of other medications have been implicated (Stochus & Allescher, 1993). Rather than preexisting esophageal dysfunction, medication-induced injury is more likely caused by inadequate fluid intake, the position of the patient when swallowing, the size of the tablet or capsule, the dissolution rate of the tablet or capsule, and the age and cognitive function of the patient.

The incidence of pill-induced esophageal injury can be greatly reduced by following simple guidelines for medication administration. Nurses, medication aides, family caregivers, and patients need to understand and appreciate the importance of taking medications correctly. The five simple steps listed in Exhibit 6–1 will ensure that once the medication is administered, it will reach the stomach as quickly as possible. In addition to avoiding injury to the esophagus, the medication must reach the stomach to start the process of dissolution and absorption, and thus the onset of drug action.

Exhibit 6–1 Medication Administration Guidelines To Reduce Risk of Esophageal Injury

---

1. Avoid taking medications **just** before lying down. Wait 5 to 10 minutes to ensure that medications have passed through the esophagus into the stomach. Taking a medication "at bedtime" means take **before** bedtime.
2. Position the bedbound patient. Elevate upper body when administering medication. Keep the patient elevated for 5 to 10 minutes.
3. Administer fluids **before** and **after** each tablet or capsule. Take several swallows before taking the medication to moisten the mouth and throat. Follow with a half to a full glass of liquid (water is preferable). Fluids will enhance the rate of dissolution of the tablet or capsule, reducing risk of focal injury.
4. Request liquid medications. Liquid medications may be available for the patient who has difficulty swallowing pills. Follow steps (1) or (2) and (3) before administering liquid medications.
5. Crush tablets or open capsules *only* with permission of the pharmacist. Crushing tablets or opening capsules may be feasible if the pill does not have an enteric coat (to prevent dissolution in the stomach) or is not designed to be long-acting. Medications mixed with food must be given **immediately** after mixing to ensure integrity of active ingredient. Follow steps (1) or (2) and (3).
6. One at a time! Patients with swallowing difficulties should take one pill at a time, following steps (1) or (2) and (3).

XEROSTOMIA

Dysphagia caused by xerostomia can be the result of impaired bolus transport due to dry mouth and mucus membranes. In a study of more than 500 patients (mean age, 70 years), those who complained of experiencing xerostomia in the morning were two to three times more likely to report that food sticks in their throats, and to experience difficulty in chewing, starting a swallow, and in swallowing than patients without xerostomia (Loesche, Bromberg, Terpenning, Bretz, Dominguez, Grossman, & Langmore, 1995). Xerostomia can also result in decreased ability to clear acid from the esophagus, thus compromising an important defense mechanism against esophagitis (Loesche et al., 1995). Patients who complain of dry mouth should be screened for medications that contribute to the problem, with the hope that the medication can be changed or discontinued (Lloyd, 1983). The use of saliva substitutes may provide some patient relief. Frequent sips of water or other beverages should be encouraged between meals. Water can be used during the meal to help swallowing. Patients may need to be specifically advised to drink fluids during the meal, particularly if they were discouraged from drinking water during meals as children.

TARDIVE DYSKINESIA

Antipsychotic drugs (Table 6–1), excluding clozapine and respiradone, cause clinically significant tardive dyskinesia (TD) in approximately 10% to 20% of all patients who take these drugs for a year. The rate may even be higher in the elderly (Baldessarini, Cole, Davis, Simpson, Tarsy, Gardos, & Preskorn, 1980; Zaratzian, 1980). TD usually involves the orofacial and lingual muscles. The syndrome can progress to the extent that patients may be unable to chew or swallow and require tube feeding. Aspiration pneumonia is another serious reported complication (Sliwa & Lis, 1993). The only treatment is prevention, by reducing exposure to these drugs. Careful monitoring for early TD symptoms, drug tapering if symptoms appear, and use of an atypical antipsychotic (respiradone, clozapine) are the most reasonable approaches to prevention in the patient who requires treatment with an antipsychotic medication.

DYSPHAGIA AND NUTRITIONAL STATUS

Patients experiencing severe dysphagia symptoms often lose weight. Medications used to treat other problems may contribute to this weight loss by decreasing a patient's appetite. Drugs can have a direct impact on food intake by causing anorexia, or they may have indirect effects, by causing an alteration in taste, nausea, and abdominal discomfort. More dramatically, antineoplastics, antivirals, and certain antibiotics may cause stomatitis, pharyngeal ulceration, or superinfection (e.g., oral candidiasis after chemotherapy). Patients who experience dysphagia as a result of antimicrobial or chemotherapy should be considered for enteral or parenteral nutrition. Table 6–5 lists common drugs that may lead to reduced food intake.

Table 6–5 Mechanisms of Drug-Induced Decrease in Food Intake

Mechanism	Medications
Anorexia	Antineoplastics, digitalis, fluoxetine, iron supplements, decongestants (pseudoephedrine), stimulants (methylphenidate), NSAIDs, potassium, theophylline, selective serotonin reuptake inhibitors (SSRIs) (Prozac, Paxil, Zoloft), buproprion (Wellbutrin), narcotic analgesics
Loss of taste	Allopurinol, antihistamines, bismuth, carbamazepine, gold compounds, griseofulvin, penicillamine
Metallic taste	captopril, lithium, potassium streptomycin

CONCLUSION

Medications may contribute to problems associated with dysphagia. A thorough review of all prescribed medications should precede or coincide with the evaluation of the patient. In some cases, adjusting the medications may improve symptoms, whereas in other cases, eliminating medications may be helpful. A complete drug history, including over-the-counter drugs, can be performed by the clinical pharmacist as part of the workup of patients with dysphagia. Lifestyle factors, such as alcohol intake, caffeine use, and smoking, also should be considered because these have been implicated in certain types of dysphagia. Special instructions on proper medication administration should be provided to all patients and their caregivers.

REFERENCES

Baldessarini, R.J., Cole, J.O., Davis, J., Simpson, G., Tarsy, D., Gardos, G., & Preskorn, S.H. (1980). Tardive dyskinesia: Summary of a task force report of the American Psychiatric Association. *American Journal of Psychiatry, 137*, 1163–1172.

Berger, K., & McCallum, R.W. (1982). Nifedipine in the treatment of achalasia. *Annals of Internal Medicine, 96*, 61–62.

Bortolotti, M., & Labo, G. (1981). Clinical and manometric effects of nifedipine in patients with esophageal achalasia. *Gastroenterology, 80*, 39–44.

Bott, S., Prakash, C., & McCallum, R.W. (1987). Medication-induced esophageal injury: Survey of the literature. *American Journal of Gastroenterology, 82*, 758–763.

Bushman, M., Dobmeyer, S.M., Leeker, L., & Permutter, J.S. (1989). Swallowing abnormalities and their response to treatment in Parkinson's disease. *Neurology, 39*, 1309–1314.

Castell, D.O. (1975). The lower esophageal sphincter: Physiologic and clinical aspects. *Annals of Internal Medicine, 83*, 390–401.

Clouse, R.E. (1993). Motor disorders. In M.H. Sleisenger, J.S. Fordtran (Eds.), *Gastrointestinal disease* (pp. 341–377). Philadelphia: W.B. Saunders Co.

Cohen, S. (1979). Motor disorders of the esophagus. *New England Journal of Medicine, 301*, 184–191.

Cohen, S. (1992). Diseases of the esophagus. In J.B. Wyngaarden, L.H. Smith, Jr., J.C. Bennett (Eds.), *Cecil Textbook of Medicine* (pp. 639–648). Philadelphia: W.B. Saunders Co.

The Diabetes Control and Complications Trial Research Group. (1993). Effect of intensive treatment of diabetes on the development and progression of long term complications in insulin-dependent diabetes mellitus. *New England Journal of Medicine, 329*, 977–986.

Diamant, N.E. (1993). Physiology of the esophagus. In M.H. Sleisenger, J.S. Fordtran (Eds.), *Gastrointestinal disease* (pp. 319–330). Philadelphia: W.B. Saunders Co.

Feinberg, M. (1993). The problems of anticholinergic adverse effects in older patients. *Drugs & Aging, 3*, 335–348.

Gelfond, M., Rozen, P., & Gilat, R. (1982). Isosorbide dinitrate and nifedipine treatment of achalasia: A clinical, manometric and radionuclide evaluation. *Gastroenterology, 83*, 963–969.

Haynes, R.C. (1990). Adrenocorticotropic hormone; adrenocortical steroids and their synthetic analogs; inhibitors of the synthesis and actions of adrenocortical hormones. In A.G. Gilman, T.W. Rall, A.S. Nies, P. Taylor (Eds.) *Goodman and Gilman's the pharmacological basis of therapeutics* (p. 1441). New York: Pergamon Press, Inc.

Haynes, R.C. (1990). Thyroid and antithyroid drugs. In A.G. Gilman, T.W. Rall, A.S. Nies, P. Taylor (Eds.) *Goodman and Gilman's the pharmacological basis of therapeutics* (p. 1376). New York: Pergamon Press, Inc.

Helm, J.F., Dodds, W.J., Pelc, J.R., Palmer, D.W., Hogan, W.J., & Teeter, B.C. (1984). Effect of esophageal emptying and saliva on clearance of acid from the esophagus. *New England Journal of Medicine, 310*, 284–288.

Higgs, R.H., Smyth, R.D., & Castell, D.O. (1974). Effect on lower-esophageal-sphincter pressure and serum gastrin. *New England Journal of Medicine, 291*, 486–490.

Kahrilas, P.J., & Hogan, W.J. (1993). Gastroesophageal reflux disease. In M.H. Sleisenger, J.S. Fordtran (Eds.), *Gastrointestinal disease* (pp. 378–401). Philadelphia: W.B. Saunders Co.

Keshavarzian, A., Iber, F.L., & Ferguson, Y. (1987). Esophageal manometry and radionuclide emptying in chronic alcoholics. *Gastroenterology, 92*, 651–657.

Keshavarzian, A., Polepalle, C., Iber, F.L., & Durkin, M. (1990). Esophageal motor disorder in alcoholics: Result of alcoholism or withdrawal? *Alcoholism, Clinical and Experimental Research, 14*, 561–567.

Klinkenberg-Knol, E.C., Festen, H.P.M., & Meuwissen, S.G.M. (1995). Pharmacological management of gastro-oesophageal reflux disease. *Drugs, 49*, 695–710.

Koller, W.C., Silver, D.E., & Lieberman, A. (Eds.). (1994). An algorithm for the management of Parkinson's disease. *Neurology, 44* (Suppl 10), S24.

Korsten, M.A., Rosman, A.S., Fishbein, S., Shlein, R.D., Goldberg, H.E., & Biener, A. (1991). Chronic xerostomia increases esophageal acid exposure and is associated with esophageal injury. *American Journal of Medicine, 90*, 701–706.

Kurlan, R., & Como, P. (1988). Drug-induced Alzheimerism. *Archives of Neurology, 45*, 356–357.

Larson, E.B., Kukull, W.A., Buchner, D., & Reifler, B.V. (1987). Adverse drug reactions associated with global cognitive impairment in elderly persons. *Annals of Internal Medicine, 107*, 169–173.

Lloyd, P.M. (1983). Xerostomia: Not a phenomenon of aging. *Wisconsin Medical Journal, 82*, 21–22.

Loesche, W.J., Bromberg, H., Terpenning, M.S., Bretz, W.A., Dominguez, B.L., Grossman, N.S., & Langmore, S.E. (1995). Xerostomia, xerogenic medications and food avoidances in selected geriatric groups. *Journal of the American Geriatrics Society, 43*, 401–407.

Marshall, J.B., Kretschmar, J.M., & Diaz-Arias, A.A. (1990). Gastroesophageal reflux as a pathogenic factor in the development of symptomatic lower esophageal rings. *Archives of Internal Medicine, 150*, 1669–1672.

Murad, F. (1990). Drugs used for the treatment of angina: Organic nitrates, calcium-channel blockers, and β-adrenergic antagonists. In A.G. Gilman, T.W. Rall, A.S. Nies, P. Taylor (Eds.), *Goodman and Gilman's the pharmacological basis of therapeutics* (p. 768). New York: Pergamon Press, Inc.

Nostrant, T.T., Sams, J., & Huber, T. (1986). Bethanechol increases the diagnostic yield in patients with esophageal chest pain. *Gastroenterology, 91*, 1141–1146.

Richter, J.E. (1993). Heartburn, dysphagia, odynophagia, and other esophageal symptoms. In M.H. Sleisenger, J.S. Fordtran (Eds.), *Gastrointestinal disease* (pp. 331–339). Philadelphia: W.B. Saunders Co.

120   DYSPHAGIA: A CONTINUUM OF CARE

Richter, J.E., Dalton, C.B., Bradley, L.A., & Castell, D.O. (1987). Oral nifedipine in the treatment of noncardiac chest pain in patients with the nutcracker esophagus. *Gastroenterology*, *93*, 21–28.

Sliwa, J.A., & Lis, S. (1993). Drug-induced dysphagia. *Archives of Physical Medicine and Rehabilitation*, *74*, 445–447.

Stochus, B., & Allescher, H.D. (1993). Drug-induced dysphagia. *Dysphagia, 8*, 154–159.

Sunderland, T., Tariot, P.N., Cohen, R.M., Weingartner, H., Mueller, E.A. (III), & Murphy, L. (1987). Anticholinergic sensitivity in patients with dementia of the Alzheimer type and age-matched controls. A dose-response study. *Archives of General Psychiatry*, *44*, 418–426.

Taylor, P. (1990). Anticholinesterase agents. In A.G. Gilman, T.W. Rall, A.S. Nies, P. Taylor (Eds.), *Goodman and Gilman's the pharmacological basis of therapeutics* (pp. 142–146). New York: Pergamon Press, Inc.

Thomas, E., Lebow, R.A., Gubler, R.J., & Bryant, L.R. (1984). Nifedipine for the poor-risk elderly patient with achalasia: Objective response demonstrated by solid meal study. *Southern Medical Journal*, *77*, 394–396.

Traube, M., Hongo, M., Magyar, L., & McCallum, R.W. (1984). Effects of nifedipine in achalasia and in patients with high-amplitude peristaltic contractions. *Journal of the American Medical Association*, *252*, 1733–1736.

Triadafilopoulos, G., Aaronson, M., Sackel, S., & Burakoff, R. (1991). Medical treatment of esophageal achalasia. Double-blind crossover study with oral nifedipine, verapamil, and placebo. *Digestive Diseases and Sciences*, *36*, 260–267.

Vitale, G.C., Cheadle, W.G., Patel, B., Sadek, S.A., Michel, M.E., & Cuschieri, A. (1987). The effect of alcohol on nocturnal gastroesophageal reflux. *Journal of the American Medical Association*, *258*, 2077–2079.

Weber, L.D., Nashel, D.V., & Mellow, M.H. (1981). Pharyngeal dysphagia in alcoholic myopathy. *Annals of Internal Medicine*, *95*, 189–191.

Wong, R.K.H., Maydonovitch, C., Gargia, J.E., Johnson, L.E., & Castell, D.O. (1987). The effect of terbutaline sulfate, nitroglycerin, and aminophylline on lower esophageal sphincter pressure and radionuclide esophageal emptying in patients with achalasia. *Journal of Clinical Gastroenterology*, *9*, 386–389.

Wright, R.A., & Penner, D.B. (1981). Myxedema and upper esophageal dysmotility. *Digestive Diseases and Sciences*, *26*, 376–377.

Zaratzian, V.L. (1980). Psychotropic drugs—neurotoxicity. *Clinical Toxicology*, *17*, 231–270.

PART **III**

Future Considerations

CHAPTER 7

Professional Education and Training

Jeri A. Logemann

This chapter is designed to: (1) outline the type of knowledge and competencies speech-language pathologists need to safely and successfully evaluate and treat patients with oropharyngeal dysphagia; (2) define the various models available to deliver this education; and (3) outline the ethical considerations of students and clinicians with little or no didactic education or practicum regarding dysphagia working in this area. This topic is currently critical, because many graduates from both undergraduate and graduate speech-language pathology programs are not adequately educated regarding dysphagia. In some cases, students or new graduates are expected to attain the knowledge and skills needed during their external practicums or while "on the job" after graduating; however, graduates usually do not have the adequate background coursework to make this on-the-job education duly meaningful and safe. Educating speech-language pathologists in the area of dysphagia is especially important because patients may die if clinicians working with dysphagic patients are not knowledgeable about the methods for assessment and treatment that reduce risks of pulmonary complications, such as pneumonia, while maintaining the highest quality of care for the patient and reducing the risk of litigation against the clinician (Martin, Corlew, Wood, Olson, Golopol, Wingo, & Kirmani, 1994).

THREE CARDINAL RULES

Safety for the clinician and the patient can be easily maintained if the clinician follows several cardinal rules regarding procedures for dysphagia evaluation and management (Exhibit 7–1). *First, swallowing should be evaluated within the context of the physiologic hierarchy of the upper aerodigestive tract* (that is, respiration is paramount for survival of the mechanism, followed by swallowing, and finally communication). The clinician should first evaluate the patient's respira-

Exhibit 7–1 Three Cardinal Rules for Dysphagia Management

---

1. Evaluate the patient in the context of the physiology of the upper aerodigestive tract:
   - respiration
   - swallowing
   - phonation
2. Administer small amounts of food during instrumental diagnosis and clinical bedside examination.
3. Do not feed patients if an unknown pharyngeal stage dysphagia is present; conduct an instrumental examination first.

---

tory status and define any breathing difficulties that may affect the patient's ability to close the airway adequately during the pharyngeal swallow (Martin, Logemann, Shaker, & Dodds, 1994). In this way, any respiratory difficulties triggered by the stress of airway closure during swallowing will be anticipated, and the physiologic mechanism will not be compromised by the evaluation of the mechanism's role and function in swallowing. A patient with severe respiratory difficulties may not be ready for a swallowing assessment. Students should have knowledge of the anatomy, physiology, and neurophysiology of respiration and speech before being educated about swallowing disorders. The knowledge of normal and abnormal swallowing then can be applied to the physiologic hierarchy of the mechanism.

Second, unless the patient is already eating orally, only very small amounts of food should be given to the dysphagic patient during any diagnostic testing and particularly during a clinical or bedside assessment. In this way, any risk of aspiration can be minimized. Procedures for maintaining patient safety should be included in the education on dysphagia diagnostic procedures (Splaingard, Hutchins, Sulton, & Chaudhuri, 1988).

Third, patients should not be fed when the clinician suspects a pharyngeal stage dysphagia but does not know the specific nature of that dysphagia. Rather, an instrumental procedure that can define the patient's pharyngeal anatomy and swallow physiology should be conducted. As a result, possible aspiration, and any risks to the dysphagic patient and the clinician will be minimized. Literature on the relationship between aspiration noted during videofluorographic procedures and the patient's risk of developing aspiration pneumonia also should be included in the education of clinicians (Martin et al., 1994; Schmidt, Holas, Halvorson, & Reding, 1994).

With these rules, clinicians can reduce their risk of liability and effectively evaluate the dysphagic patient's oropharyngeal mechanism for its capability to maintain safe oral intake or to return to safe oral intake. A clinician with an inadequate educational background may not understand the physiologic hierarchy of the upper aerodigestive tract or the importance of eliminating as much risk as possible for the patient. Clinicians who are not educated in dysphagia may succumb to the pressures of supervisors who instruct them to provide therapy to patients who cannot be expected to benefit. Clinicians who were not adequately educated also may defer to nurses or physicians less knowledgeable about evaluation and treatment of swallowing and their accompanying risks, and who recommend oral intake for the patient without having adequate information about the patients' swallowing capabilities. Or, a poorly trained clinician may feed a patient at another professional's request when obvious signs of patient intolerance of the feeding, such as coughing, gurgly voice, and increased chest congestion are present. It is critical for the speech-language pathologist working in the area of dysphagia to: (1) maintain independent decision-making, (2) make recommendations and treatment plans based on physiologic information, and (3) not follow the suggestions of other professionals less informed in swallowing physiology. A clinician who is well educated in normal swallowing physiology and dysphagia is the key to restoration of safe and efficient oral intake in the oropharyngeal dysphagic patient.

This chapter will examine the various options for providing education in dysphagia including undergraduate education, coursework, practica at the master's level, and doctoral education in evaluation and treatment of swallowing disorders and normal swallow physiology. Models for continuing education will be discussed. Continuing education in dysphagia is critically needed because clinicians who graduated from programs that did not offer this coursework need to gain knowledge in the area, and new information on normal swallow physiology as well as evaluation and treatment procedures is rapidly increasing. Finally, dysphagia study groups are also important for clinicians to maintain clinical skills in evaluation and treatment of dysphagia.

KNOWLEDGE AND COMPETENCIES NEEDED TO WORK IN THE AREA OF DYSPHAGIA

The speech-language pathologist working in the area of dysphagia needs to have a large, integrated knowledge base as well as many attributes and skills or competencies to work efficiently and safely with a wide range of dysphagic patients. The knowledge base required to be successful as a swallowing therapist is more broad and deep than that necessary in any other area within the speech-language pathologist's domain. To evaluate and treat dysphagic clients effectively, the speech-language pathologist must understand the normal anatomy and physiology of the upper aerodigestive tract, a wide range of disease processes and types of congenital and acquired damage to the central nervous system, and the structures of the upper aerodigestive tract itself which can cause dysphagia (Dodds, Taylor, Stewart, Kern, Logemann, & Cook, 1989; Doty, 1968; Logemann, 1983). The swallowing therapist also must be knowledgeable in the recovery effects and degenerative processes characteristic of each of these disorders (Lazarus, Logemann, Kahrilas, & Mittal, 1994; Lazarus & Logemann, 1987; Robbins, Logemann, & Kirshner, 1986; Robbins, Hamilton, Lof, & Kempster, 1992; Sonies, 1995). In addition, information on normal anatomy and physiology of respiration and swallowing at various ages, from birth through old age, must be integrated with information on disease processes, and structural and neurologic damage for the clinician to distinguish normal from abnormal swallowing and define optimal treatment strategies (Jacob, Kahrilas, Logemann, Shah, & Ha, 1989; Kahrilas & Logemann, 1993; Robbins et al., 1992; Tracy, Logemann, Kahrilas, Jacob, Kobara, & Krugler, 1989.

The speech-language pathologist working in the area of dysphagia must maintain up-to-date knowledge about the various imaging procedures that can be applied to the assessment of anatomy and physiology of the upper aerodigestive tract during deglutition, as well as about the nonimaging instrumental procedures, such as electromyography and manometry, that can be used in evaluating and treating deglutition (Dodds, Logemann, & Stewart, 1990; Dodds, Stewart, & Logemann, 1990; Donner, 1988; Ergun, Kahrilas, & Logemann, 1993; Langmore, Schatz, & Olsen, 1988; Perlman, Luschei, & DuMond, 1989; Reimers-Neils, Logemann, & Larson, 1994; Shawker, Sonies, Hall, & Baum, 1984). The clinician must know what each of these instrumental procedures does and does not reveal about the anatomy and physiology of the upper aerodigestive tract during respiration and swallowing, and their applicability to various populations by age and disorder (Sonies, 1995). The dysphagia clinician must be able to interpret and integrate the results of various assessments, make therapy and management recommendations based on these results, and communicate these results to the patient, family, attending physician, and other members of the health care team in a clear and effective manner. The speech-language pathologist must be familiar with all of the risks inherent in evaluation and treatment of swallowing disorders and ways to minimize these risks. The swallowing therapist must be familiar with all of the various treatment regimens and management procedures for dysphagia including compensatory strategies; exercise programs; swallow maneuvers; surgical procedures applied to the upper aerodigestive tract; prosthetic approaches to improving oropharyngeal swallowing; effects of medication(s) on oropharyngeal swallowing, including drugs that may worsen the patient's swallowing and medications that may improve swallow physiology; and dietary and nutritional interventions. The speech-language pathologist must be knowledgeable about the various costs of each evaluation and rehabilitation procedure they conduct, and able to compare these costs with those of procedures offered by other specialists, including surgical procedures and intraoral prosthetics. The clinician must be familiar with and competent when practicing counseling techniques for patients and their significant others, as well as knowledgeable about the legal and ethical issues involved when treating patients with dysphagia and counseling families regarding living wills and other types of advance directives. The speech-language pathologist working with dysphagic patients also must be skilled in supervising support personnel who are needed, in some settings, to carry out the maintenance therapy programs or the feeding recommendations. The speech-language pathologist also must understand how to advocate on behalf of the patient within any setting where dysphagic individuals may be receiving services and have special needs.

OVERVIEW OF EDUCATIONAL MODELS REGARDING DYSPHAGIA

Because swallowing is a critical biologic function of the upper aerodigestive tract and that anywhere from 30% to 90% of a speech-language pathologist's time in health care settings, and an increasing percentage in educational settings, may be spent evaluating and treating dysphagic patients, in-depth education in normal swallow anatomy and physiology, as well as education about techniques for assessment and treatment of the patient, should be critical parts of the undergraduate and master's level curriculum in speech-language pathology, and integrated into the entire curriculum. Unfortunately, only approximately one-half of the educational programs in speech-language pathology currently offer some education in dysphagia to their master's level students, and many of these are devoting only a part of a course to the topic. This is not adequate to educate clinicians to work effectively with dysphagic patients.

Dysphagia educational programs should begin at the undergraduate level with basic science coursework and proceed in an integrated, sequential fashion to the master's level. The master's curriculum should include both a course in dysphagia and dysphagia-related information in other courses concentrating on disorders causing both communication and swallowing problems (Special Interest Division Newsletter—Swallowing and Swallowing Disorders [dysphagia], 1995). The master's level curriculum also should include practica experiences with patients who have dysphagia of various etiologies. There is also need for doctoral education in dysphagia to produce university faculty who are able to teach the previously described coursework. Doctoral level professionals are needed to conduct research in normal and abnormal swallowing.

Once master's level students have completed their graduate curriculum and have received their certificate of clinical competence, continuing education in dysphagia is necessary to maintain their knowledge base at the "cutting edge" of the profession, as well as their competencies in conducting evaluation and treatment procedures. In addition to continuing education, dysphagia study groups are one method for maintaining skills needed in assessment and treatment of swallowing disorders, such as reading or interpreting radiographic studies. Each of these various educational levels will be discussed in more detail.

Undergraduate Education in Dysphagia: Integration of Dysphagia Education into the Undergraduate Curriculum

Most undergraduate educational programs in speech-language pathology include a great deal of information on normal anatomy, physiology, and neurophysiology, as well as on normal processes of speech, language, hearing, etc. These basic science courses should include an in-depth discussion of the anatomy and physiology of normal respiration and swallowing behavior of infants and adults, including the elderly (Sonies, Baum, & Shawker, 1984; Sonies, Parent, Morrish, & Baum, 1988; Robbins et al., 1992; Tracy et al., 1989). The range of normal swallowing behaviors within each age group should be discussed and emphasized, because there is a growing body of knowledge regarding the systematic changes in normal oropharyngeal swallow physiology based upon characteristics of the food swallowed including the bolus volume (Kahrilas, Dodds, Dent, Logemann, & Shaker, 1988; Kahrilas & Logemann, 1993; Dodds et al., 1989; Logemann, Kahrilas, Cheng, Pauloski, Gibbons, Rademaker, & Lin, 1992), viscosity, taste, and temperature (Lazarus, Logemann, Rademaker, Kahrilas, Pajak, Lazar, & Halper, 1993), as well as regarding the effects of voluntary control on swallow physiology (Bisch, Logemann, Rademaker, Kahrilas, & Lazarus, 1994; Kahrilas, Logemann, & Gibbons, 1992). This information could be included as a unit in the course on anatomy and physiology of the "vocal tract" or upper aerodigestive tract. A section devoted to swallow and respiratory neurophysiology also could be included in the coursework on the innervation and neurophysiology of this region. The integration of swallowing, respiration, and speech production should be emphasized.

In addition to these basic science courses, departments of communication sciences often offer survey courses of disorder areas at the undergraduate level. A section on dysphagia should be included within these survey courses. There is a growing body of knowledge regarding the nature of swallowing disorders resulting from various types of structural and/or neurologic damage, whether acquired or congenital or pediatric or adult, that also should be introduced in these survey courses. This information may be presented in a case-history format presenting detailed information on the overall diagnostic process of the patient including respiratory, swallowing, and speech function, and treatment planning and implementation.

It is critical for clinicians to gain problem-solving skills while at the undergraduate level and expand on these skills while at the graduate level, using information from the courses on normal anatomy, physiology, neurology, and neurophysiology, as well as from the survey courses of disorders. Problem-solving skills are important in developing each clinician's thought processes in the evaluation and treatment of any disorder, but particularly in dysphagia, which requires the clinician to draw upon a broad knowledge base in designing and implementing the assessment and treatment plan for the management of the patient's dysphagia in the context of their disease process, family constellation, and other related factors. At the undergraduate level, students often memorize information, not applying it to the context of patient care until they reach the graduate level. Then, as graduate students, they have, unfortunately, forgotten much of this information that they had memorized and either they must review in-depth or, more problematically, they may not have the basic information that they need "at their finger-tips" when managing patients. In management of dysphagia, the clinician must have a day-to-day working knowledge of the anatomy, physiology, and neurophysiology of the mechanism. Without that kind of basic science information integrated into their thinking, clinicians will not be able to interpret imaging studies of the mechanism or understand the patient's swallowing disorder(s), and select assessment and treatment strategies appropriately. At the undergraduate level, time devoted to the development of problem-solving skills and utilization of basic science information to solve theoretical patient problems will directly impact the student's ability to solve clinical problems confronting them while at the master's level and during daily life as a clinician managing patients with swallowing disorders.

Master's Level Curriculum

The master's level curriculum should include a course in dysphagia that lasts one semester or one quarter of the school year, taught and tested on a competency basis. This course should include and integrate information on the set of behaviors defined as normal swallowing physiology and the characteristics of swallow in normal individuals of all ages. The relationship between swallowing and respiration should be discussed. If possible, the course should be taught in a problem-solving manner such that the student is required to use the information on normal processes and various types of neurologic, anatomic, or physiologic damage to plan evaluation and treatment for swallowing dysfunction in a particular patient. For example, students may be presented with the case of an 85-year-old patient with Parkinson's disease and dysphagia. To define the dysphagia in this individual, the students would need to: (1) compare the patient's swallowing physiology derived from a diagnostic procedure (i.e., instrumental data collection procedure such as videofluoroscopy) with similar data from the swallow physiology of an 85-year-old "normal" individual; and (2) define those aspects of the patient's swallow physiology that result from Parkinson's disease (which requires that the students know the typical swallowing disorders seen in patients with Parkinson's disease, as well as the range of disorders seen); (3) compare the information described in (2) with the physiology of a "normal" 85-year-old subject; and (4) determine whether other diagnostic procedures are needed to fully understand the patient's swallowing disorder(s) and design an effective management plan. In this way, students can learn how to use and integrate the information they have gained on normal and abnormal swallowing physiology, various disease processes, and techniques of assessment and treatment. In this example, students also would need to know the therapy techniques that are helpful for a patient with the swallowing disorders resulting from Parkinson's disease. They would need to know whether there are special issues involved in the management of dysphagia in patients with Parkinson's disease—in particular, the nature of the treatment that works best or does not work well for this type of patient.

At the master's level, the course on dysphagia should require that students become competent in conducting and interpreting radiographic studies of swallowing and videoendoscopic studies of swallowing, and be familiar with the kinds of data that can be derived from scintigraphy, ultrasound, electromyography, and manometry (Logemann, 1993). These kinds of skills can be developed using videotapes of patient diagnostic studies that are available for such training. The course also should include information on the various types of structural damage, medical and neurologic diseases, and neurologic damage that can cause dysphagia, and the kinds of swallowing disorders typically seen in these populations (Lazarus & Logemann, 1987; Robbins, 1987; Robbins & Levine, 1988). When discussing these kinds of special populations, it is critical to discuss the effects of the disease processes or damage on the entire function of the upper aerodigestive tract, including respiration and communication, to consider swallowing within the context of the full range of function of the mechanism, and to consider any special effects each type of damage or disease has on recovery and/or compensatory ability.

The master's level course in dysphagia also should provide students with experience in clinical decision-making and writing reports. Clinical decision-making includes selecting strategies to assess particular patients, followed by treatment procedures and their rationales. It is critical that students and clinicians be able to describe the scientific rationale for all diagnostic and treatment procedures they use. This is what distinguishes a clinician from a technician. Students also should be provided with experiences in writing diagnostic reports (and daily chart notes) for both assessment and treatment. The ways in which students describe the results of the procedures they use and their rationales will contribute to their success or failure as a clinician. Report writing should include description of the swallowing disorder(s) observed in a particular patient, the patient's response to compensatory and/or therapy procedures, recommendations for oral and/or nonoral feeding, the kind of treatment to be initiated, and the schedule for assessment, if applicable. These types of skill-building activities within the graduate curriculum would lead directly to practicum.

Practicum in Dysphagia at the Master's Level

If students have received competency-based education, including experiences in report writing and therapy planning, they should be ready for their practicum where they should receive in-depth, hands-on experiences with dysphagic patients. A practicum in dysphagia should be closely supervised, as in all practica, and should provide the student with experiences in assessing and treating swallowing disorders, as well as counseling patients and their significant others. The practica should include patients with dysphagia resulting from as many different etiologies as possible to provide the student with experience in managing patients of different ages and disorder types.

Practice sites should be selected carefully to give the student the widest range of experiences possible. Students should be involved in "bedside" or clinical assessments of dysphagic patients, and in videofluoroscopic and other assessments of oropharyngeal swallow, as well as in report writing regarding these cases to build competence. They should have opportunities to treat inpatients and outpatients with dysphagia and to use a full range of treatment strategies. If possible, they should have opportunities to at least observe manometric studies of oropharyngeal swallowing, endoscopic examinations of oropharyngeal swallow, and other instrumental procedures. Experience with designing clinical recommendations, and counseling patients and families about these recommendations also should be included. Discussion of ethical issues concerning recommendations for nonoral feeding and patients who are unwilling to comply with these recommendations should be included. Whenever possible, students should have an opportunity to work with patients representing a wide age range, from infants through the elderly.

Inclusion of Dysphagia Information in Other Coursework at the Master's Level

Courses in motor-speech disorders, head and neck cancer, voice disorders, cerebral palsy or pediatric neurologic disorders, and geriatrics should all include sections on dysphagia. Again, as in the course specifically devoted to dysphagia (evaluation and treatment of swallowing disorders), the full range of effects of these disorders on the upper aerodigestive tract should be emphasized. Within the discussion of each of the specific types of swallowing disorders, the therapy and diagnostic techniques that are most appropriate and those that are most inappropriate for a particular population should be carefully defined, along with rationales for these differences.

Doctoral Education in Dysphagia

With the increasing emphasis on dysphagia in the clinical practice of speech-language pathologists, there is need for faculty at the doctoral level who can teach courses in dysphagia, and related anatomy and physiology of the upper aero-digestive tract. There is also a need for more research on normal swallow physiology and on the various disorders that affect oropharyngeal swallowing. There is need for more opportunities for doctoral education and postdoctoral study in dysphagia. Topics for research by doctoral and postdoctoral students include examination of relationships between respiration and swallowing, and between communication disorders and dysphagia, as well as normal swallow physiology and neurophysiology.

Continuing Education

As long as students graduate from master's degree programs with an inadequate education in dysphagia, there will be significant need for continuing education opportunities regarding all of the aspects of dysphagia management including normal swallow physiology, evaluation and treatment techniques, and needs of special populations. In addition, even those students who graduate from master's programs with a strong education in dysphagia need to maintain their skills, as well as remain familiar with the latest developments in dysphagia management. Therefore, even those individuals who have an excellent background in the areas of normal swallowing and dysphagia will need to remain on the cutting edge of patient care by taking advantage of opportunities in continuing education.

Continuing education can provide an ever-expanding knowledge base for the working clinician. It allows the clinician to update knowledge as new findings are published. Continuing education also can be used to build skills. Much of the information on dysphagia and development of most of the competencies required to treat this disorder area involve processing visual information that can be presented in continuing education courses with video projection of case studies. Entire days of continuing education activity can focus on the interpretation of and treatment planning devised from videofluorographic studies, endoscopic studies, measurement of outcomes from various treatment procedures, etc. An important topic throughout the education of clinicians is measurement of efficacy and outcomes. Measurement of efficacy involves defining measurable differences in patient performance with and without a particular swallowing procedure, or from one time to another. Definition of the outcomes of therapy involves identifying changes in patient behavior that most importantly reduce cost, such as returning a patient to oral intake or reducing the need for nursing care by eliminating nonoral feedings other than thin liquids. Eliminating aspiration associated with certain foods, which enables the patient to take those kinds of foods orally, is another significant quality of life outcome that also reduces cost of care. Educational programs for clinicians should emphasize the various techniques for measuring outcome, efficacy, and cost.

DYSPHAGIA STUDY GROUPS

Dysphagia study groups help clinicians to maintain their skills. Reading and interpreting radiographic studies is a skill that can diminish if not used regularly. Dysphagia study groups that meet regularly enable clinicians to maintain their skill levels by providing them with the opportunity to read and interpret video-fluorographic studies from other clinicians and discuss these relative to treatment decisions and recommendations regarding oral/nonoral intake. Dysphagia study groups also provide the opportunity to review recent literature and discuss its clinical implications. Also, continuing education workshop experiences could be shared with other clinicians through study groups. In any community where three or four clinicians are working in the area of dysphagia, study groups that can reinforce each clinician's knowledge and skills, as well as challenge their thinking about difficult cases could be organized easily.

ETHICAL AND LEGAL CONSIDERATIONS

Many ethical issues arise during the evaluation and treatment of dysphagic patients. Some of these stem from graduates who have had no coursework or practical (well-supervised) experience in dysphagia taking jobs that involve a substantial amount of dysphagic therapy. University faculty should counsel students in this regard. Clinicians should not accept positions in facilities where they will be treating dysphagic patients until they have gained the necessary knowledge and skills. Another major ethical issue arises from the implementation of advance directives by staff, family, and patient. These types of directives and their relationship to the patient's diagnosis and to the speech-language pathologist's involvement should be discussed in the dysphagia education program.

All educational experiences in the area of dysphagia should include discussions of ethical issues and how these issues should be handled. Students and clinicians should also refer to the Code of Ethics of the American Speech-Language-Hearing Association and published "Issues in Ethics" statements for guidance.

Methods for Successful Inservicing and Relating to Other Professionals

Dysphagia education programs should include information on successful and productive ways to involve other professionals in the care of the dysphagia patient. Effective procedures and available materials for providing inservice education on dysphagia to other professionals should also be described.

CONCLUSION

Overall, there are many methodologies available for expanding the knowledge and skills of students and clinicians in the area of dysphagia. Maintaining skills and competencies is critical in this area for the patient to achieve and maintain good health. A clinician who is not up-to-date in his or her knowledge or skills can cause significant harm to a dysphagic patient. Clinicians who are overly confident about their skills also can do harm, thinking they can do more with bedside work, for example, than is feasible or safe. It is important that graduate education programs instill in their students the need for continuing their education after graduation through a variety of means, many of which have been discussed in this chapter.

Dysphagia can be a rewarding clinical area in which to work if the clinician is knowledgeable about the anatomy and physiology of the normal and abnormal upper aerodigestive tract, and if the clinician has a healthy respect for his or her limitations in assessing and understanding this mechanism from a bedside approach. Clinicians with less knowledge and experience often will take their direction from a supervisor or physician who has inadequate knowledge in dysphagia and will proceed to feed a particular dysphagic patient, despite lack of knowledge about the patient's oropharnygeal physiology. The inexperienced clinician may even proceed to feed a patient in response to a physician's suggestion, despite obvious signs (such as coughing) that the patient has significant swallowing difficulty. Clinicians should have a healthy respect for what they do and do not know and not proceed in an area in which they have little knowledge. Clinicians who are well educated and competent in dysphagia management can be highly successful and ethical in evaluating and treating dysphagic patients.

REFERENCES

Bisch, E.M., Logemann, J.A., Rademaker, A.W., Kahrilas, P.J., & Lazarus, C.L. (1994). Pharyngeal effects of bolus volume, viscosity and temperature in patients with dysphagia resulting from neurologic impairment and in normal subject. *Journal of Speech and Hearing Research, 37*, 1041–1049.

Dodds, W.J., Logemann, J.A., & Stewart, E.T. (1990). Radiological assessment of abnormal oral and pharyngeal phases of swallowing. *American Journal of Roentgenology, 154*, 965–974.

Dodds, W.J., Stewart, E.T., & Logemann, J. (1990). Physiology and radiology of the normal oral and pharyngeal phases of swallowing. *American Journal of Roentgenology, 154*, 953–963.

Dodds, W.J., Taylor, A.J., Stewart, E.T., Kern, M.K., Logemann, J.A., & Cook, I.J. (1989). Tipper and dipper types of oral swallows. *American Journal of Roentgenology, 153*, 1197–1199.

Donner, M. (1988). The evaluation of dysphagia by radiography and other methods of imaging. *Dysphagia, 1*, 49–50.

Doty, R.W. (1968). Neural organization of deglutition. In C.F. Code (Ed.), *Handbook of physiology, alimentary canal* (Sec. 5, Vol. 4)(pp. 1861–1902). Washington, DC: American Physiology Society.

Ergun, G.A., Kahrilas, P.J., & Logemann, J.A. (1993). Interpretation of pharyngeal manometric recordings: Limitations and variability. *Diseases of the Esophagus, 6,* 11–16.

Jacob, P., Kahrilas, P., Logemann, J., Shah, V., & Ha, T. (1989). Upper esophageal sphincter opening and modulation during swallowing. *Gastroenterology, 97,* 1469–1478.

Kahrilas, P., Dodds, W., Dent, J., Logemann, J., & Shaker, R. (1988). Upper esophageal sphincter function during deglutition. *Gastroenterology, 95,* 52–62.

Kahrilas, P.J., & Logemann, J.A. (1993). Volume accommodations during swallowing. *Dysphagia, 8,* 259–65.

Kahrilas, P.J., Logemann, J.A., & Gibbons, P. (1992). Food intake by maneuver: An extreme compensation for impaired swallowing. *Dysphagia, 7,* 155–159.

Langmore, S.E., Schatz, K., & Olsen, N. (1988). Fiberoptic endoscopic examination of swallowing safety: A new procedure. *Dysphagia, 2* (4), 216–219.

Lazarus, C., & Logemann, J.A. (1987). Swallowing disorders in closed head trauma patients. *Archives of Physical Medicine and Rehabilitation, 68,* 79–87.

Lazarus, C.L., Logemann, J.A., Kahrilas, P.J., & Mittal, B.B. (1994). Swallow recovery in an oral cancer patient following surgery, radiotherapy, and hyperthermia. *Head & Neck, 16* (3), 259–265.

Lazarus, C.L., Logemann, J.A., Rademaker, A.W., Kahrilas, P.J., Pajak, T., Lazar, R., & Halper, A. (1993). Effects of bolus volume, viscosity and repeated swallows in non-stroke subjects and stroke patients. *Archives of Physical Medicine and Rehabilitation, 74,* 1066–1070.

Logemann, J.A. (1983). *Evaluation and treatment of swallowing disorders.* Austin, TX: Pro-Ed.

Logemann, J.A. (1993). *A manual for videofluoroscopic evaluation of swallowing* (2nd ed.) Austin, TX: Pro-Ed.

Logemann, J.A., Kahrilas, P.J., Cheng, J., Pauloski, B.R., Gibbons, P.J., Rademaker, A.W., & Lin, S. (1992). Closure mechanisms of the laryngeal vestibule during swallow. *American Journal of Physiology, 262* (*Gastrointestinal and Liver Physiology, 25*), G338–G344.

Martin, B.J., Corlew, M., Wood, H., Olson, D., Golopol, L., Wingo, M., & Kirmani, N. (1994). The association of swallowing dysfunction and aspiration pneumonia. *Dysphagia, 9,* 1–6.

Martin, B.J.W., Logemann, J.A., Shaker, R., & Dodds, W.J. (1994). Coordination between respiration and swallowing: Respiratory phase relationships and temporal integration. *Journal of Applied Physiology, 76* (2), 714–723.

Perlman, A.L., Luschei, E.S., & DuMond, C.E. (1989). Electrical activity form the superior pharyngeal constrictor during reflexive and non-reflexive tasks. *Journal of Speech and Hearing Research,* 749–754.

Reimers-Neils, L., Logemann, J.A., & Larson, C. (1994). Viscosity effects on EMG activity in normal swallow. *Dysphagia, 9,* 101–106.

Robbins, J.A. (1987). Swallowing in ALS and motor neuron disorders. *Neurologic Clinics, 5,* 213–229.

Robbins, J., & Levine, R. (1988). Swallowing after unilateral stroke of the cerebral cortex: Preliminary experience. *Dysphagia, 3,* 11–17.

Robbins, J., Hamilton, J.W., Lof, G.L., & Kempster, G.B. (1992). Oropharyngeal swallowing in normal adults of different ages. *Gastroenterology, 103,* 823–829.

Robbins, J., Logemann, J., & Kirshner, H. (1986). Swallowing and speech production in Parkinson's disease. *Annals of Neurology*, *19*, 283–287.

Schmidt, J., Holas, M., Halvorson, K., & Reding, M. (1994). Videofluoroscopic evidence of aspiration predicts pneumonia and death but not dehydration following stroke. *Dysphagia*, *9*, 7–11.

Shawker, T., Sonies, B., Hall, T., & Baum, G. (1984). Ultrasound analysis of tongue, hyoid and larynx activity during swallowing. *Investigative Radiology*, *19*, 82–86.

Sonies, B.C. (1991). Instrumental procedures for dysphagia diagnosis. *Seminars in Speech and Language*, *12* (3), 185–198.

Sonies, B.C. (1995). Progression of oral-motor and swallowing symptoms in the post-polio syndrome. The Post-Polio Syndrome: Advances in Pathogenesis and Treatment. *Annals of the New York Academy of Sciences*, *753*, 87–95.

Sonies, B.C., Baum, B.J., & Shawker, T.H. (1984). Tongue motion in elderly adults: Initial in situ observations. *Journal of Gerontology*, *39* (3), 279–283.

Sonies, B., Parent, L., Morrish, K., & Baum, G. (1988). Durational aspects of the oral-pharyngeal phase of swallow in normal adults. *Dysphagia*, *3*, 1–10.

Special Interest Division Newsletter—Swallowing and Swallowing Disorders (Dysphagia Issues in Educational Preparation)(1995), Div. 13, Vol 4 (2), 2–10.

Splaingard, M., Hutchins, B., Sulton, D., & Chaudhuri, J. (1988). Aspiration in rehabilitation patients: Videofluoroscopy vs. bedside clinical assessment. *Archives of Physical Medicine and Rehabilitation*, *69*, 637–640.

Tracy, J., Logemann, J., Kahrilas, P., Jacob, P., Kobara, M., & Krugler, C. (1989). Preliminary observations on the effects of age on oropharyngeal deglutition. *Dysphagia*, *4*, 90–94.

CHAPTER 8

Application of Instrumental Procedures to the Evaluation and Treatment of Dysphagia

Adrienne L. Perlman

The purpose of examining for dysphagia is first to determine if dysphagia is present, and if so, to diagnose the features and estimate the severity of the problem; this requires a full understanding of the physiology of deglutition since it is the physiological aspects of the swallow that are assessed. As a result of the examination findings, the clinician then decides what treatment to recommend. When a patient is first seen because of signs of dysphagia, the assessment generally begins with the clinical examination, also known as the "bedside" examination. At this time, the examiner obtains the necessary information regarding the patient's medical diagnosis, general health, living conditions, cognitive and speech/language history, and history of dysphagia. A thorough case history and clinical examination are imperative to the decision-making process and should not be overlooked. Specific discussion of the clinical examination is provided elsewhere (Perlman, Langmore, Milianti, Miller, Mills, & Zenner, 1991; Schulze-Delrieu & Miller, 1996) and, therefore, is not discussed in this chapter.

Although the clinical examination provides important information to assist with the decision-making process, various dysphagic signs cannot be adequately diagnosed during this examination. In fact, it has been shown that only 42% to 66% of the dysphagia patients who experience aspiration may be identified during a clinical examination (Splaingard, Hutchins, Sulton, & Chaundhuri, 1988; Linden, Kuhlemeier, & Patterson, 1993). The presence of other signs of dysphagia, for example residue in the valleculae or pyriform sinuses, cannot be identified during a clinical examination; those signs are highly related to aspiration (Perlman, Booth, & Grayhack, 1994). Consequently, for the purpose of objective and complete diagnosis, imaging and measurement techniques are required.

Because of the need to visualize the pharynx and larynx, the most frequently used method for diagnosis of swallowing disorders is the videofluoroscopic (also called videofluorographic) examination (VFE) of swallow function. The VFE provides information on the oral and pharyngeal stages of swallowing and can follow the bolus into the esophagus so that the radiologist or gastroenterologist can assess esophageal function.

Although the VFE is considered the "gold standard" for assessing the oral and pharyngeal stages of the swallow, other examinations provide important information regarding specific aspects of these two stages of deglutition. The other procedures can assist with medical diagnosis, as well as with determination of the features and severity of the problem, and often can help with determination of treatment recommendations. The procedures generally are used as adjuncts to the VFE. The more frequently used adjuncts to examination are the fiberoptic endoscopic examination of swallowing (FEES^{SM}) and ultrasound; however, electromyography, electroglottography, and the measurement of respiration during swallowing are useful instrumental techniques that aid with answering specific questions regarding the swallow. This chapter will discuss the application of each of these methods of assessment and treatment.

VIDEOFLUOROSCOPY

VFE is the most widely used and, in most instances, the most appropriate tool for an initial examination. The primary reason for performing a videofluoroscopic examination is to assess the physiology of the swallow. From the outcome of the examination, the clinician can determine: (1) if patients can continue safe oral intake, (2) if patients can progress from their present method of nourishment to oral intake, (3) if patients are likely to meet their nutritional requirements with oral nourishment and, (4) if it is advisable to implement alternative methods of nutrition. With VFE, the clinician is able to determine the duration and, to a certain extent, the completeness of bolus transit as well as obtain information regarding the movement patterns of most of the oral and pharyngeal structures associated with deglutition. Additionally, the symmetry of bolus transport, penetration of radio-opaque material into the laryngeal vestibule, and tracheobronchial aspiration can be observed. During this examination, a clinician often can determine if changes in bolus volume or viscosity, or in a patient's posture, can result in a safer, more efficient swallow.

Even if aspiration does not occur during the examination, one can roughly estimate the likelihood of the occurrence of aspiration by studying the video observations (Perlman et al., 1994). A major strength of the videofluoroscopic assessment

---

Note: FEES^{SM} is a service mark of Susan Langmore, PhD.

is that the underlying cause of aspiration generally can be identified from the video observations, (Kahrilas, Logemann, S, & Ergun, 1992). The primary disadvantage of the VFE is the need to limit the amount of radiation exposure to which the patient is subjected. Another disadvantage is the difficulty of transporting some patients to facilities that have videofluoroscopic equipment.

Videofluoroscopic Equipment

With the proper equipment, a clinician can determine the severity of the swallowing problem, communicate information that can assist with diagnosis and management of the medical problem to the patient's physicians, and make valid treatment decisions. In many institutions, some of the equipment is kept in the radiology service (Figure 8–1) and the remainder in the speech pathology service (Figure 8–2). For example, the radiology suite would contain an SVHS recorder, a videomonitor, a microphone, and a time-date generator. The speech pathology service would have a compatible videorecorder and videomonitor, and a videoprinter. An additional option is to use a video measuring gauge. Along with an available spreadsheet, this gauge allows the clinician to perform a quantitative analysis of structural displacement (Perlman, VanDaele, & Otterbacher, 1995). There is good rationale for using each component.

To obtain the best possible resolution from a videorecorder without spending an extraordinary amount of money, the choice of machine should be a commercial-quality, 4-track SVHS with a jog and shuttle and frame lock. This will permit the examiner to review the examination at variable decreased speeds or frame-by-frame, which is necessary for accurate interpretation.

When an SVHS recorder is used, a high resolution monitor is needed to show the greater number of lines per inch that is produced with the SVHS recorder. A picture-reduction control on the videomonitor is useful. Picture reduction makes the image clearer, but it should not be used when recording. This control is useful when viewing the recorded tape after the study.

To record running dialogue, a microphone is needed. This audio record on the videotape helps the clinician remember what bolus volume or viscosity the patient was swallowing, and what comments the patient may have made regarding sensations or concerns, and permits the clinician to provide descriptive discussion of the patient's performance during examination. The style of microphone depends upon the layout of the examining room. Microphones that attach to clothing can cause one to trip on the cord when walking around the room; but, if that is the only available method for assuring that speech is recorded, then one should use the clip-on microphone and just be careful. A correctly placed stationary microphone is preferred.

A time-date generator is important because it imprints a timing code on the videotape. This allows for accurate assessment of all temporal measurements in-

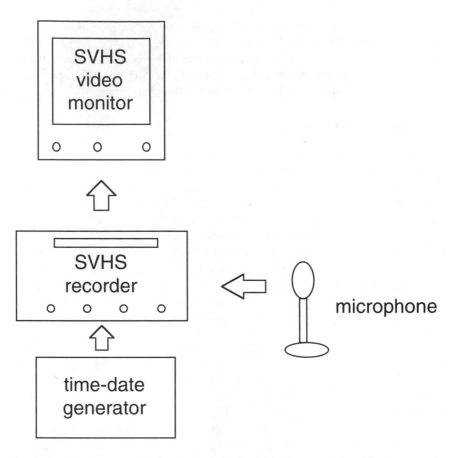

Figure 8–1 Equipment configuration for recording video images during videofluoroscopic examination of swallowing function.

cluding the duration of the oral preparatory phase, the extent of the delay in triggering the pharyngeal stage of the swallow, the duration of pharyngeal transit, the duration of upper esophageal sphincter opening, and, when observed, the duration of esophageal transit. Time-date generators can provide information that is accurate to one hundredth of a second (some models display to the thousandth). The digital readout of the tape recorder displays time in seconds and, therefore, is inadequate for most of the purposes listed previously.

Attaching a black and white print from a videoprinter to a clinical report can prove to be useful in communicating with a physician. Because the physician may

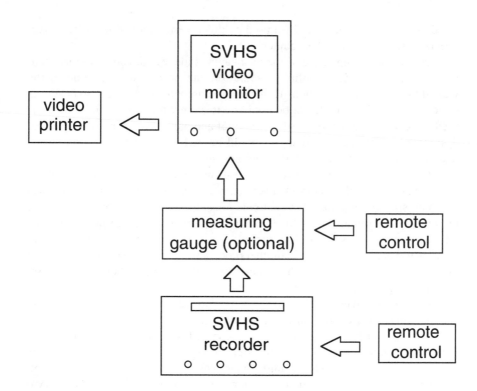

Figure 8–2 Equipment configuration for analysis of video images from the videofluoro-scopic examination of swallowing function.

read only the impressions and recommendations portion of the videofluoroscopic report, a print of the video image showing, for example, the extent of aspiration or of hypopharyngeal stasis can convey the importance of the clinical findings.

One last piece of equipment that the clinician may want to consider is a video measuring gauge (For-A). This has been found to be an effective, and reasonably easy way of quantifying the extent of movement of important structures such as the hyoid bone (Perlman et al., 1995). The clinician must have a computer and a spreadsheet program (Excel or Lotus) to interpret the findings.

Several texts discuss the interpretation of the videofluoroscopic procedure (Logemann, 1993; Perlman, Lu, & Jones, 1996). Consequently, test interpretation will not be discussed in this chapter. However, it is important to remember that the speech-language pathologist performs this examination to assess oral and pharyn-geal swallowing *function* (that is, physiology). The functional aspects of VFE are listed in the copy of the VFE form used by this investigator and included as Appendix 8–A at the end of this chapter.

Once the underlying cause of the dysphagia is identified, compensatory techniques and variations in bolus presentation can be tested at the end of the videofluoroscopic examination. However, the amount of radiation exposure is critical and the VFE should not be used as a treatment tool nor should it be overused by lengthy examinations. If a structural anomaly, neoplasm, or esophageal dysfunction is suspected, the study should be performed in conjunction with a radiologist or at least reviewed by a radiologist.

Whereas the VFE procedure permits the examiners to view the entire swallowing event, from mouth to stomach, the remaining techniques that will be discussed are more specific regarding the anatomic areas they examine. This is the major reason why it is usually advisable to begin the instrumental assessment using the VFE. Once the entire swallow is observed, the speech-language pathologist (SLP) is in a better position to decide if another procedure should be performed as part of the initial assessment or if another procedure can be used as follow-up, and if so, which other procedure(s) to select.

There are times when a VFE cannot be performed first. For example, a patient may be frail or too ill to be transported to the radiology service, or the consult may have arrived shortly before a patient is discharged from the hospital and there is insufficient time to schedule the procedure before the patient goes home. If the VFE cannot be performed as the initial examination, the FEES may be an acceptable procedure because it can detect premature spillover, pharyngeal and laryngeal residue, and often can indicate the presence of laryngeal penetration.

Example of Use of the Videofluoroscopic Procedure

R.W. was a 64-year-old female who experienced a stroke approximately 5 days before she was referred to the SLP for examination. On clinical examination, it was noted that the patient was severely aphasic and exhibited signs of oral and pharyngeal weakness. The patient had an inconsistent wet cough and her voice quality was characterized as "wet hoarse." R.W. had been fed by nasogastric tube since her hospital admission but there was family pressure to remove the tube.

The patient was seen for a VFE of swallowing function. Results of the examination revealed a moderately severe dysphagia characterized by a severe delay in initiation of the pharyngeal stage of the swallow, reduced hyoid and laryngeal elevation, diffuse hypopharyngeal stasis, and aspiration before and after the swallow. The tape of this examination was shown to the patient's family. Viewing the tape helped them to understand the need for the nasogastric tube and eliminated their requests to have it removed. Subsequently, the patient was started on swallowing therapy as well as language therapy. The patient's daughter helped R.W. to practice her exercises each day when she came to visit. Because she had been given adequate information to understand the dysphagia condition and the purpose of the assigned swallowing therapy exercises, the daughter provided helpful assistance to the SLP.

FIBEROPTIC ENDOSCOPIC EXAMINATION OF SWALLOWING

Videolaryngoscopy with flexible or rigid endoscopes has been performed routinely by otolaryngologists and SLPs for assessment of laryngeal function during voice production. While the physician is the only professional who is licensed to render a medical diagnosis, the properly trained SLP is qualified to assess laryngeal function. The fiberoptic endoscopic examination of swallowing is an extension of the techniques used for flexible endoscopy in the assessment of voice production. Consequently, an SLP who has been trained to do flexible fiberoptic laryngoscopy and who has expertise in the assessment of swallowing could be easily trained to perform this procedure.

Both the Dysphagia Special Interest Group and Voice Special Interest Group of the American Speech-Language-Hearing Association are in the process of developing guidelines for training clinicians to perform laryngeal endoscopy. Until those guidelines are confirmed, it is up to the SLP who is interested in developing expertise in FEES to receive training from an experienced user of FEES, either an SLP or otolaryngologist. The SLP should continue training until the mentor determines that the trainee is qualified to independently perform and interpret the technique.

The equipment used for assessment of swallowing function is the same as that used for flexible videolaryngoscopy; consequently, if the clinician is already performing laryngeal endoscopy with a flexible fiberscope, no equipment cost is involved in beginning to practice this procedure. The equipment consists of a flexible fiberoptic endoscope, camera, appropriate light source, SVHS recorder and monitor, and a microphone (Figure 8–3). The technique is well described elsewhere (Langmore, Schatz, & Olsen, 1988; Langmore, Schatz, & Olson, 1991; Bastian, 1991; Langmore & McCulloch, 1996).

Basically, the fiberscope is inserted transnasally and a traditional velar and laryngeal examination is performed. Then the endoscope is moved until it is situated above the valleculae. When appropriate, the patient receives various bolus volumes and viscosities, and the events that occur before and after the swallow can be observed. If water is given, it is advisable to color the fluid with a drop of blue or green food coloring; if it is not colored, it is somewhat difficult to see the fluid well. Some clinicians prefer to use milk rather than water. Because there is no radiation associated with this procedure, the larynx and pharynx can be observed for extended periods. If the patient is not at risk, he or she can receive various

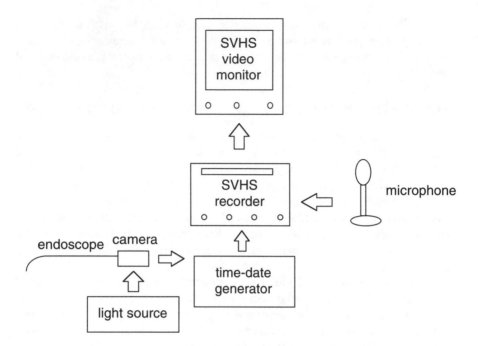

Figure 8–3 Equipment configuration for recording the fiberoptic endoscopic examination of swallowing.

---

types of food and varying bolus volumes; the patient as well as the clinician can observe the video monitor; thus, when appropriate, biofeedback can be provided during or after the procedure. If the patient has excessive secretions or gives an indication during bedside examination of an absent or weak swallow, the structures can be observed during a swallow attempt without introducing any food or liquid. In such cases, it is advisable to place a small drop of food coloring on the patient's tongue. This procedure may be difficult for agitated or noncompliant patients, and may require a topical nasal anesthetic. A protocol for the FEES examination is presented in Appendix 8–B.

Timing of the movements of the bolus, larynx, and epiglottis, and a description of endoscopic observations have been reported (Perlman & VanDaele, 1993). These data can serve as guidelines for more objective assessment with FEES. Those temporal values are reported in Table 8–1 and will be discussed more completely in the section on ultrasound in this chapter.

The major limitations of the FEES are that the oral stage cannot be observed and the pharyngeal and laryngeal view is obliterated during the swallow. Additionally, the clinician must develop expertise in performing and interpreting the procedure, and if the equipment is not available, there is a significant cost for the SVHS recorder, high resolution monitor, time-date generator, microphone, light source, and endoscope. Lastly, the patient must be cooperative; for example, a patient with a moderate to severe movement disorder such as Huntington's chorea or dystonia can be studied with fluoroscopy, but it can be extremely difficult and often inadvisable to assess that patient with endoscopy. Furthermore, the procedure is contraindicated for patients who have bleeding disorders and for fragile patients.

There are, however, instances when videofluoroscopy cannot be performed and FEES may serve as the primary examination tool. Data indicating how well this procedure can serve as a replacement for the videofluoroscopic procedure is not yet available. However, FEES is a second tool that gives an excellent view of pharyngeal and laryngeal structures, except during the swallow when the picture is obliterated by the contraction of the pharyngeal muscles and tongue base retraction. As stated earlier, the absence of radiation makes it an excellent therapeutic tool for providing visual biofeedback to some patients.

Kidder, Langmore, and Martin (1994) state that "several rare but potential risks and complications" are associated with the procedure which either the examining clinician or another qualified individual who is in close proximity must be prepared to treat; these include vasovagal reaction, laryngospasm, nasal hemorrhage, and adverse medication reaction. When performing any invasive procedure, equipment for resuscitation and persons qualified to perform cardiopulmonary resuscitation (CPR) should be readily available. In hospital settings or medical clinics, the availability of qualified assistance, if needed, is not a problem; but the problem does need to be considered and addressed in environments such as nursing homes and university speech and hearing clinics. Because some registered nurses are qualified to insert nasogastric tubes, those individuals may be qualified to serve as medical backup if a physician is not in-house. However, the dependence upon a nurse for medical emergency backup should be approved by the patient's physician before the procedure is performed.

Example of Use of the FEES Procedure

J.D. is a 64-year old male who had undergone a partial laryngectomy approximately 4 weeks previously and was in the early stages of radiation therapy. The patient had been evaluated with a VFE 2 weeks after surgery. At that time, it was learned that, among other findings, there was significant pyriform sinus residue and silent aspiration.

The patient came to see the speech-language pathologist and requested another examination; he stated that he thought his swallow was just fine and that he wanted to begin eating. The clinician suspected that the patient was unable to accurately estimate the safety of the swallow because of the loss of sensation to the affected area. Consequently, the clinician contacted the patient's physician and explained the situation. The SLP stated that she would like to perform a FEES and have the patient view the videotape during the examination. The physician agreed to this request for a follow-up examination, and the FEES was performed by the SLP.

After inserting the endoscope, a drop of green food coloring was placed on the patient's tongue. Because of the excessive aspiration visualized during the VFE just 2 weeks before, the clinician assumed that the problem would probably remain. Consequently, she began the study without giving the patient a food or liquid bolus. By seating the patient so that he could see the video monitor along with the clinician, it was possible for the clinician to explain the occurrence of events to the patient and to have him see his saliva penetrating the larynx. The patient could also see the secretions that were sitting in the pharynx, and the clinician could explain that if the patient could not manage his secretions, he could not yet manage food. While the fiberscope was inserted, therapy techniques such as the Mendelsohn maneuver were practiced in an effort to improve the opening of the upper esophageal sphincter. The patient was able to see the lack of effect of these techniques during the procedure and he agreed to remain NPO with the agreement that further testing was to be performed at a later time.

ULTRASOUND

As described in chapter 9, ultrasound images are produced by high-frequency sound waves that are reflected and then received by the ultrasound transducer and subsequently assembled into a video image. Soft tissue such as the tongue allows for good passage of the ultrasound waves; the interface between two surfaces, such as the tongue and the palate, present themselves as a change in acoustic impedance, and waves are reflected from that interface (Sonies, 1991). However, bone is too dense to permit passage of the ultrasound waves and so the waves are reflected off the bone; because of this, the acoustic shadow from the hyoid bone can be tracked even though the structure itself cannot be visualized. Thus, tissues can be differentiated by their ability to reflect the sound waves, and because the mouth is mostly soft tissue surrounded by air, ultrasound is effective for examining the oral stage and the initiation of the pharyngeal stage of the swallow.

Experienced clinicians can use a 5 MHz linear transducer and visualize the larynx during adduction and elevation. Any ultrasound system produced during the last 8 years can be used. The small, wand-like transducer is placed at the level of the thyroid notch and moved in small increments until the image is clear. To correctly interpret the test results correctly, the examiner must be able to differentiate the images of the true and false vocal folds by watching phonation and humming; at first, this requires practice. The clinical application of this technique for the assessment of aspiration has not yet been validated.

Table 8–1 shows the means and standard deviations of observations that were made during swallowing of nonmeasured boluses in a simultaneous videoendoscopy and sagittal plane ultrasound study (Perlman & VanDaele, 1993). All measurements were made relative to the first view (endoscopic) of the bolus at the level of the base of tongue/valleculae. The superscript "u" indicates that the measure was made from the ultrasound image. The temporal measures of the hyoid bone displacement were found to be compatible with measurements reported in other ultrasound investigations (Sonies, Parent, Morrish, & Baum, 1988). Also, the duration of the endosocopic image that was obscured because of image whiteout was 469 milliseconds; that value is in agreement with the 443 milliseconds reported from the oropharyngeal pressure wave during swallowing (Perlman, Schultz, & VanDaele, 1993). Thus, it appears that the whiteout is primarily the result of pharyngeal constrictor contraction; tongue base retraction may contribute somewhat to the increased pressure as well as to the image whiteout.

In a recent paper (Sapper & Sonies, 1995), ultrasound was found to be correlated to VFE on certain features of the swallow. If a delay of 450 milliseconds or greater was found on the ultrasound measure of hyoid elevation and tongue flattening, then the VFE observation of pharyngeal pooling could be predicted in 90% of the cases. Associations such as this are valuable tools in patient assessment.

Table 8–1 Results from Simultaneous Ultrasound and Fiberoptic Endoscopic Examinations of Swallowing

	OAA	IEM	IHM^u	CP	MHD^u	IHD^u	OP	RE	RHB^u	Total
Mean time (ms)	−416	−136	−75	205	350	668	674	758	927	1328
SD	174	163	151	64	111	98	82	63	91	192

All time is in milliseconds and is relative to the first view of the bolus, which was observed endoscopically as it flowed over the base of the tongue. Negative numbers indicate activities that occurred before the first view of the bolus. OAA = onset of arytenoid adduction, IEM = initial epiglottic movement, IHM = initial hyoid movement, CP = close of the pharynx, MHD = maximum hyoid deflection, IHD = initial hyoid descent, OP = opening of the pharynx, RE = return of the epiglottis, RHB = return of the hyoid to baseline.

Source: Reprinted with permission by Singular Publishing Group, Inc. from A.L. Perlman and D.J. VanDaele, Simultaneous videoendoscopic and ultrasound measures of swallowing. *Journal of Speech-Language Pathology*, vol. 1, pp. 223–232. © 1995 Singular Publishing Group, 401 West "A" Street, Suite 235, San Diego, California 92101-7904, 1-800-521-8545.

In a useful tutorial, anatomic sections of the tongue and floor of mouth were correlated with the anatomy as visualized by ultrasound (Gritzmann & Fruhwald, 1988). The material presented in that paper is fundamental to interpretation of the ultrasound image. As with other examination procedures, it is important to have an examination format and record of performance. Appendix 8–C contains a checklist for the ultrasound assessment of swallowing.

The major advantage of ultrasound is that the procedure is noninvasive and risk-free; consequently, if the clinician has ascertained that a patient's problems are oral, this procedure can be repeated multiple times with no risk to the patient. A child or infant can be studied safely (Casas, Kenny, & McPherson, 1994) and, if needed, positioned in the parent's lap for comfort. Also, the examination can be performed without the need to give the patient a test bolus. If a bolus is given, it can be any food or liquid. Additionally, ultrasound can be used for biofeedback during treatment (Shawker, Stone, & Sonies, 1984).

The major disadvantages are that the view is essentially limited to the oral cavity and oropharynx, and minimal information is provided regarding the presence of vallecular or pyriform sinus residue, laryngeal penetration, laryngeal displacement, or aspiration. Thus, unlike videofluoroscopy or endoscopy, the information that is obtained is very specific. The following procedures that are described are also specific regarding the information they provide.

Unfortunately, the application of ultrasound to treatment has not been extensively discussed in the literature. The technique has strong possibilities for treatment with infants and children as well as adults, and for speech as well as swallowing (Casas et al., 1994). The ability to see the motion and position of the tongue and the hyoid bone during motion with no negative radiation effects make this an excellent medium to consider for therapy.

Example of Use of the Ultrasound Procedure

P.L. was a female patient who had experienced a stroke at age 56 years. After her stroke, the patient had no involvement of her lower extremities, but did have unilateral weakness of the right upper extremity. She exhibited some language deficits but was able to follow two-step commands and to communicate her thoughts reasonably well. There was evidence of both oral and pharyngeal weakness on swallow. She was able to decrease the extent of her aspiration to inconsistent, trace aspiration only if she performed serial swallows with each bolus and if she avoided viscous foods with pudding consistencies and solids. On close examination of the VFE, it became apparent that much of the problem with swallowing related to weakness in the muscles of the floor of the mouth and tongue.

The patient was seen for swallowing therapy and encouraged to do the assigned exercises on her own at least two times during the day. The extent of muscle shortening in the submental (below the chin) coronal plane was measured during the first ultrasound session, and the relative change in the extent of muscle shortening was measured weekly. Additionally, the extent of hyoid bone displacement in the sagittal plane was measured weekly. The video image was explained to the patient and she was instructed in how to interpret the tongue and hyoid movements; thus, studying the video image became a method by which she could confirm her own improvement in swallowing. Although she could use the ultrasound machine only when the clinician was there to work with her, the ability to see the extent of muscle contraction during her therapy session provided an added incentive to work hard when she practiced on her own, and provided her with the instant feedback needed to learn to control the swallow.

ELECTROMYOGRAPHY

Human skeletal muscle is comprised of muscle fibers which, depending upon the muscle, can vary from approximately 10 to 100 μm in diameter and from a few millimeters up to 30 cm in length. Each muscle contains thousands of fibers, and each fiber, which is the structural unit of muscle activity, is part of a motor unit. The motor unit consists of the cell body, located in the central nervous system; its axon; the neuromuscular junctions; and the muscle fibers that are innervated by the axon.

When a motoneuron is activated, all the muscle fibers it innervates become activated. There are as few as three and as many as 2,000 skeletal muscle fibers in a motor unit. Muscles that require fine movement control, such as eye or laryngeal muscles, have few fibers per motor unit, whereas muscles of gross movement such as the leg muscles have large numbers of fibers per unit.

The release of acetycholine at the neuromuscular junction results in a flow of current that spreads to the interior of the muscle fiber. This causes the release of calcium ions that then initiate the chemical events that cause the muscle fiber contraction. As the number of activated motoneurons increases, the number of contracting muscle fibers increases; this results in increased strength of the muscle contraction.

When a muscle fiber or group of fibers contract, a small electrical signal is produced. The signal from the muscle can be picked up by an antenna that, in this instance, is called an electrode. Because these signals are so small, it is necessary to greatly amplify them; generally, this amplification is done in two steps. The signal then can be recorded or input directly into a computer where the analysis will be performed. The signal can be displayed on either an oscilloscope or a computer monitor. A speaker that permits the electromyographer to hear the electromyographic (EMG) signal produced by the contracting muscle is strongly recommended; the audio signal provides important qualitative information, for example the approximate distance from the motor units and the condition of the electrodes or the contracting muscles.

Figures 8–4, 8–5, and 8–6 are representative of the electromyographic signals from the thyroarytenoid muscle of a normal adult subject. The first figure is representative of a single firing from a single motor unit; the second figure shows a train of firings from a motor unit as they occurred over a period of 400 ms; and the last figure is the gross EMG when there is activity from many motor units during a swallow.

Two general types of electrodes, surface and intramuscular, can receive electromyographic signals. Intramuscular electrodes can be either needle electrodes or hooked-wire, and surface electrodes can be either flat surface or suction. For research in speech or swallowing, the bipolar hooked-wire electrode is generally the most appropriate type of electrode; the suction electrode (Tanaka, Palmer, & Siebens, 1986) is appropriate for some studies. However, for clinical applications

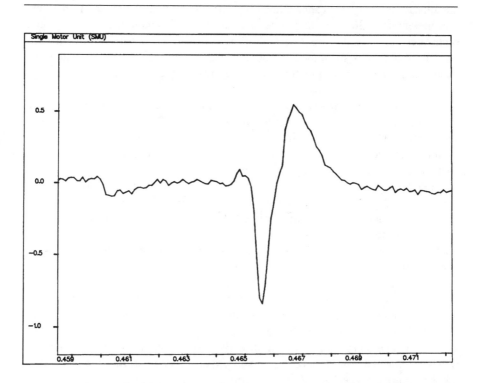

Figure 8–4 Electromyographic recording from a single motor unit. *Source:* Reprinted with permission from A.L. Perlman, *Dysphagia*, vol. 8, pp. 351–355, © 1993, Springer-Verlag.

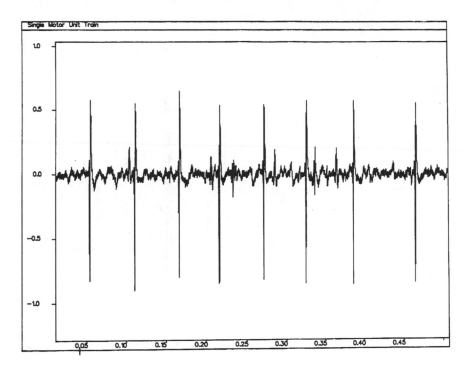

Figure 8–5 Train of firings from a single motor unit. *Source:* Reprinted with permission from A.L. Perlman, *Dysphagia*, vol. 8, pp. 351–355, © 1993, Springer-Verlag.

(such as biofeedback), a clinician almost always would use bipolar surface electrodes. When placed correctly, the surface electrodes can be used for biofeedback from the muscles close to the skin surface such as the orbicularis oris, the submental complex, or the thyrohyoid muscles. The surface electrodes are inclined to receive electrical signals from a reasonably large field; therefore, activity is likely to be recorded from muscles other than those of particular interest.

The absolute values of the amplitudes of EMG signals in two different treatment sessions cannot be compared; nor can the absolute values of two different muscles be compared. That is because the amplitude is related to many factors, including how close the electrode is placed relative to a motor unit, and one cannot place the electrode in exactly the same place each time a procedure is performed. For that reason, one must compare performances across times of measurement using relative amplitudes.

For diagnosis of neuromuscular disease, neurologists often prefer to use electromyography. Using the techniques described by various researchers (Gay,

152   DYSPHAGIA: A CONTINUUM OF CARE

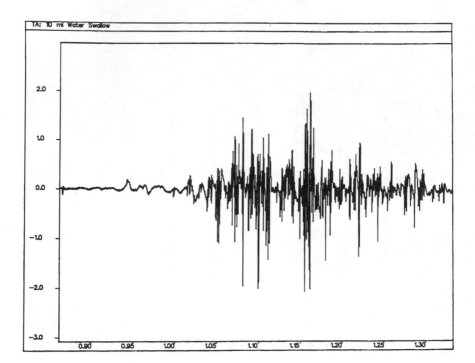

Figure 8–6 Gross EMG from the throarytenoid muscle during a 10 ml water swallow. *Source:* Reprinted with permission from A.L. Perlman, *Dysphagia*, vol. 8, pp. 351–355, © 1993, Springer-Verlag.

Hirose, Strome, & Sawashima, 1972; Hirano, Ohala, & Vernard, 1969; Thumfart, 1988; Perlman, Luschei, & DuMond, 1989), one can also verify oral, laryngeal, or pharyngeal muscle paralysis. Although not all otolaryngologists perform electromyography, many have developed expertise in electromyographic analysis of laryngeal and pharyngeal muscles. Cooper and Perlman (1996) provide an in-depth discussion of the use of EMG in the study of swallowing.

It is important that a clinician who decides to use EMG has a thorough understanding of this procedure; otherwise, it is easy to misinterpret the EMG output. Various textbooks on the subject are available. The textbook by Basmajian and DeLuca (1975) is probably the most commonly used reference; but, as with any other complicated technique, one should read more that one textbook before first using this procedure.

Example of Use of the EMG Procedure

J.F. is a 72-year-old male who was in very good health until he suffered a stroke which left him with severe dysphagia and a breathy voice quality. The patient did not have a swallow; consequently, if any food or liquid entered the pharynx, it remained there until aspirated or coughed out. Before coming to our clinic, the patient had been previously treated with a pharyngeal myotomy, which was totally ineffective because the major underlying problem had not been one of cricopharyngeal hypertonicity. Rather, his problem was due to the inability to elicit a swallow.

Rigid endoscopic examination of the larynx (transorally, not transnasally, as in FEES) had been performed earlier and revealed an inability to close the glottis during phonation; there appeared to be some movement of only one arytenoid. The endoscopic examination also revealed that the hypopharynx was filled with secretions; additionally, the patient aspirated his secretions during the laryngeal examination. Obviously, it was important to understand the underlying pathology of the swallow. Did the patient not swallow because of severe weakness or was there complete paralysis of the pharyngeal and laryngeal muscles? The only way to differentiate the two was to conduct bilateral EMG. Bipolar hooked-wire electrodes were inserted into the superior pharyngeal constrictor and into the vocal folds.

Electromyographic examination confirmed a total paralysis on one side of the pharynx and larynx, and some weak motor unit activity on the contralateral side. The weak movement was interpreted as a sign of possible regeneration of one side; consequently laryngeal and pharyngeal exercises were initiated.

ELECTROGLOTTOGRAPHY

The electroglottograph (EGG) is a noninvasive instrument that, when modified at the factory, can be used to assess the temporal aspects of laryngeal elevation during swallowing. The necessary equipment for assessment during swallowing consists of the EGG and an instrument to observe the signal output, such as a storage oscilloscope or a computer monitor. Although EGGs can have either one or two pairs of electrodes for the assessment of swallowing, we have had the most success with those that have two pairs (Glottal Enterprises, Syracuse, NY).

If one wishes to purchase an EGG for use in swallowing assessment or treatment, it is necessary to advise the company of your intent. The electrodes that are used only for assessing vocal fold contact area during voice production are standard with the instrument and are different from those that are used for assessing voice and/or swallowing. The modifications made by the manufacturer are minor and easily provided, but the customer must request the alterations. Following modification, the EGG can still be used for analysis of vocal fold movement during phonation.

Although electroglottography has been used for some time in the study of laryngeal function during phonation, application of the EGG to the study of swallowing has been recent (Sorin, McClean, Ezerzer, & Fishbein, 1987; Perlman & Liang, 1991; Perlman & Grayhack, 1991; Schultz, Perlman, & VanDaele, 1994). In the assessment of the temporal aspects of laryngeal motion, the disc electrodes are placed externally on opposite sides of the neck. The electrodes on one side serve as a transmitter and send out a high frequency, constant-amplitude signal. The electrodes on the opposite side receive the signals after they have been modified by the change in laryngeal position during the swallow. The change in position is represented by a change in the magnitude of the signal as it passes through the neck.

The following figure (Figure 8–7) shows the appearance of the EGG signal from the two electrodes. Notice that they are essentially the reverse of one another; this is because during the swallow, the input signal going through one electrode will become greater and the signal going through the other will become less. This is due to the change in the ability to conduct the signal through muscle and cartilage versus that which is going through the airspace of the subglottal region; because the anatomy is different between each pair, the signals cannot be identical.

The duration of the EGG signal representing laryngeal movement has been reported to be an average of 1.1 seconds (Schultz et al., 1994). Given this information, it is possible to use the EGG as a biofeedback method for training the patient in using the Mendelsohn maneuver, a treatment technique that results in an increased duration of laryngeal elevation.

Example of Use of the EGG Procedure

B.B. was a 57-year-old male who was experiencing post-polio syndrome that had resulted in weakness of the pharyngeal and laryngeal muscles. As a result, he experienced fatigue during mealtime with subsequent choking as well as an intermittent (but frequent) change in voice quality. On VFE, it was noted that hyoid and laryngeal elevation were of short duration and limited in excursion. Subsequently, test material remained in the valleculae and pyriform sinuses after the swallow. During the VFE examination, attempts were made to instruct the patient in how to perform a Mendelsohn maneuver. When performed correctly, the patient was able to clear the pharynx with two to three swallows; however, he could not perform this maneuver consistently.

The patient was taken to the speech pathology department and connected to the EGG. Output from the EGG was displayed on the computer monitor using CODAS (DATAQ Instruments, Akron, OH). Within less than 5 minutes, the patient was consistent in his ability to perform the Mendelsohn maneuver and also was able to associate the characteristics of the EGG output with the sensation of muscle fatigue. When fatigue was evident, the patient stopped eating for a few minutes, rested, and then was able to return with good laryngeal elevation.

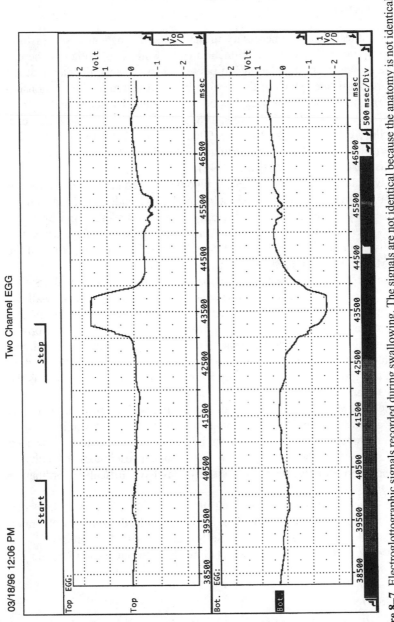
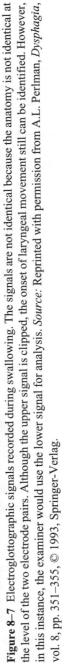

Figure 8–7 Electroglottographic signals recorded during swallowing. The signals are not identical at the level of the two electrode pairs. Although the upper signal is clipped, the onset of laryngeal movement still can be identified. However, in this instance, the examiner would use the lower signal for analysis. *Source:* Reprinted with permission from A.L. Perlman, *Dysphagia,* vol. 8, pp. 351–355, © 1993, Springer-Verlag.

SIMULTANEOUS MEASURES OF RESPIRATION AND SWALLOWING

There are times when it is necessary to determine if a patient is successfully managing respiratory function in conjunction with swallowing. Although there is little in the literature on the relationship between these events, the data that are available are consistent. Much of the recent clinical research on the relationship between deglutition and swallowing has been performed by Selley and his colleagues (Selley, Flack, Ellis, & Brooks, 1989a; Selley, Flack, Ellis, & Brooks, 1989b; Selley, Ellis, Flack, & Brooks, 1990a; Selley, Flack, Ellis, & Brooks, 1990b; Parrott, Selley, Brooks, Lethbridge, Cole, Flack, Ellis, & Tripp, 1992; Selley, Ellis, Flack, Bayliss, & Pearce, 1994).

In a study of 12 healthy normal subjects who were given graduated volumes of water (3, 10, 20 ml) while simultaneous submental EMG, endoscopy, and plethysmography were performed, the investigators reported that respiration was halted before the onset of laryngeal elevation. Apnea was approximately 1 second in duration and expiration resumed nearly 0.50 second before the completion of the swallow (Martin, Logemann, Shaker, & Dodds, 1994).

In agreement with the previously mentioned investigators, Smith et al. (Smith, Wolkove, Colacone, & Kreisman, 1989) concluded that among adults, swallowing is almost exclusively an expiratory activity. Their study used plethysmography and submental EMG. During their investigation, seven adult males performed 271 resting swallows, as well as when eating and drinking, and only two swallows occurred during inspiration. Continued work needs to be performed with children of varying age groups to ascertain if they have the same patterns or if this is the result of maturation.

Evidence suggests that coordination of respiration with swallowing is not as consistent among individuals with certain disorders, including cerebral palsy, stroke, and motoneuron disease. Also, it can be suspected that because of the need to breathe more often, the patient who is experiencing respiratory difficulty or who has chronic obstructive pulmonary disease may have difficulty coordinating the two events.

Because of the need for more research in this area, our laboratory has been working on the development of a portable, reasonably priced, computer integrated device that, like the system used by Selley et al. (1990b), can serve as a noninvasive method for assessing the relationship between respiration and deglutition.

CONCLUSION

Although VFE of oral and pharyngeal swallowing function provides the most complete information relating to swallowing function, this technique may not adequately meet all the needs of a particular patient or patient population. The intent of this chapter was to provide clinicians with alternative techniques that can be applied to answer particular clinical questions. The choice of instrumental swallowing technique depends upon: (1) the diagnostic and treatment questions that need to be answered, (2) the environment in which the patient is to be evaluated, (3) the health status of the particular patient, and (4) the clinician's level of training and expertise. All four of these variables must be considered when determining the appropriate methodologies for assessing a particular patient. In most cases, the VFE should precede any other diagnostic procedure.

The purposes and limitations of videofluoroscopy, flexible fiberoptic endoscopy, ultrasound, electromyography, electroglottography have been described, and measurement of the temporal association between respiration and swallowing has been addressed. Examples of the application of these procedures to patient care were presented. Additionally, the Appendixes provide examples of forms for assessment of swallowing function with videofluoroscopy, flexible fiberoptic endoscopy, and ultrasound. Although not clinically useful at this time, it is likely that magnetic resonance imaging (MRI) will become fast enough to also serve as a diagnostic tool for some aspects of swallowing. Because of its excellent resolution of soft tissue structures, rapid MRI may provide clinicians with another dynamic and complete procedure to evaluate oropharyngeal physiology. We can only guess what other diagnostic procedures will become part of the armamentarium of the dysphagia clinician.

REFERENCES

Basmajian, V., & DeLuca, C. (1975). *Muscles Alive* (5th ed.). Baltimore: Williams & Wilkins Company.

Bastian, R. (1991). Videoendoscopic evaluation of patients with dysphagia: An adjunct to the modified barium swallow. *Otolaryngology—Head and Neck Surgery, 104*, 339–350.

Casas, M., Kenny, D., & McPherson, K. (1994). Swallowing/ventilation interactions during oral swallow in normal children and children with cerebral palsy. *Dysphagia, 9*, 40–46.

Cooper, D.S., & Perlman, A.L. (1996). Electromyography in the functional and diagnostic testing of deglutition. In A.L. Perlman & K. Schulze-Delrieu (Eds.), *Deglutition and its disorders: anatomy, physiology, clinical diagnosis and management.* San Diego, CA: Singular Publishing Group.

Gay, T., Hirose, H., Strome, M., & Sawashima, M. (1972). Electromyography of the intrinsic laryngeal muscles during phonation. *Annals of Otolaryngology, 81*, 401–409.

Gritzmann, N., & Fruhwald, F. (1988). Sonographic anatomy of tongue and floor of the mouth. *Dysphagia, 2*, 196–202.

Hirano, M., Ohala, J., & Vernard, W. (1969). The function of laryngeal muscles in regulating fundamental frequency and intensity of phonation. *Journal of Speech and Hearing Research, 12*, 616–628.

Kahrilas, P., Logemann, J., S, L., & Ergun, G. (1992). Pharyngeal clearance during swallow: A combined manometric and videofluoroscopic study. *Gastroenterology, 103*, 128–136.

Kidder, T.M., Langmore, S.E., & Martin, B.J.W. (1994). Indications and techniques of endoscopy in evaluation of cervical dysphagia: Comparison with radiographic techniques. *Dysphagia, 9*, 256–261.

Langmore, S.E., Schatz, K., & Olsen, N. (1988). Fiberoptic endoscopic examination of swallowing safety: A new procedure. *Dysphagia, 2*, 216–219.

Langmore, S.E., Schatz, K., & Olson, N. (1991). Endoscopic and videofluoroscopic evaluations of swallowing and aspiration. *Annals of Otology, Rhinology, and Laryngology, 100*, 678–681.

Langmore, S.E., & McCulloch, T. (1996). Endoscopic examination of the pharynx and larynx and of the pharyngeal stage of the swallow. In A.L. Perlman & K. Schulze-Delrieu (Eds.), *Deglutition and its disorders: anatomy, physiology, clinical diagnosis and management.* San Diego, CA: Singular Publishing Group.

Linden, P., Kuhlemeier, K., & Patterson, C. (1993). The probability of correctly predicting subglottic penetration from clinical observations. *Dysphagia, 8*, 170–179.

Logemann, J.A. (1993). *Manual for the videofluorographic study of swallowing* (2nd ed.). Austin, TX: Pro-Ed.

Martin, B., Logemann, J., Shaker, R., & Dodds, W. (1994). Coordination between respiration and swallowing: respiratory phase relationships and temporal integration. *Journal of Applied Physiology, 76*, 714–723.

Parrott, L.C., Selley, W.G., Brooks, W.A., Lethbridge, P.C., Cole, J.J., Flack, F.C., Ellis, R.E., & Tripp, J.H. (1992). Dysphagia in cerebral palsy: A comparative study of the Exeter dysphagia assessment technique and a multidisciplinary assessment. *Dysphagia, 7*, 209–219.

Perlman, A.L., Booth, B.M., & Grayhack, J.P. (1994). Videofluoroscopic predictors of aspiration in patients with oropharyngeal dysphagia. *Dysphagia, 9*, 90–95.

Perlman, A.L., & Grayhack, J.P. (1991). Use of the electroglottograph for measurement of temporal aspects of the swallow: Preliminary observations. *Dysphagia, 6*, 88–93.

Perlman, A.L., Langmore, S., Milianti, F., Miller, R., Mills, H., & Zenner, P. (1991). Comprehensive clinical examination of oropharyngeal swallowing function: Veterans administration procedure. *Seminars in Speech and Language, 12*, 246–254.

Perlman, A.L., & Liang, H. (1991). Frequency response of the Fourcin electroglottograph and measurement of temporal aspects of laryngeal movement during swallowing. *Journal of Speech and Hearing Research, 34*, 791–795.

Perlman, A.L., Lu, C., & Jones, B. (1996). Examination of the oral cavity, pharynx, and esophagus by static and by dynamic X-ray studies. In A.L. Perlman & K. Schulze-Delrieu (Eds.), *Deglutition and its disorders: anatomy, physiology, clinical diagnosis and management.* San Diego, CA: Singular Publishing Group.

Perlman, A.L., Luschei, E.S., & DuMond, C.E. (1989). Electrical activity from the superior pharyngeal constrictor during reflexive and nonreflexive tasks. *Journal of Speech and Hearing Research, 32*, 749–754.

Perlman, A.L., Schultz, J.G., & VanDaele, D.J. (1993). Effects of age, gender, bolus volume, and bolus viscosity on oropharyngeal pressure during swallowing. *Journal of Applied Physiology, 75*, 33–37.

Perlman, A.L., & VanDaele, D.J. (1993). Simultaneous videoendoscopic and ultrasound measures of swallowing. *Journal of Medical Speech-Language Pathology, 1*, 223–232.

Perlman, A.L., VanDaele, D.J., & Otterbacher, M. (1995). Quantitative assessment of hyoid bone displacement from video images during swallowing. *Journal of Speech and Hearing Research*, *38*, 579–585.

Sapper, D.S. & Sonies, B.C. (1995). Comparison of the timing of swallowing events using ultrasound and videofluoroscopy. Presented at the Dysphagia Research Society, McLean, VA.

Schultz, J., Perlman, A.L., & VanDaele, D.J. (1994). Laryngeal movement, oropharyngeal pressure, and submental muscle contraction during swallowing. *Archives of Physical Medicine and Rehabilitation*, *75*, 183–189.

Schulze-Delrieu, K.S. & Miller, R.M. (1996). Clinical Assessment of Dysphagia. In *Deglutition and Its Disorders: Anatomy, Physiology, Clinical Diagnosis and Management*, A.L. Perlman & K. Schulze-Delrieu (Eds.), San Diego, CA: Singular Publishing Group.

Selley, W.G., Ellis, R.E., Flack, F.C., Bayliss, C.R., & Pearce, V.R. (1994). The synchronization of respiration and swallow sounds with videofluoroscopy during swallowing. *Dysphagia*, *9*, 162–167.

Selley, W.G., Ellis, R.E., Flack, F.C., & Brooks, W.A. (1990a). Coordination of sucking, swallowing, and breathing in the newborn: Its relationship to infant feeding and normal development. *British Journal of Disorders of Communication*, *25*, 311–327.

Selley, W.G., Flack, F.C., Ellis, R.E., & Brooks, W.A. (1989a). Respiratory patterns associated with swallowing: Part 1. The normal adult pattern and changes with age. *Age and Ageing*, *18*, 168–172.

Selley, W.G., Flack, F.C., Ellis, R.E., & Brooks, W.A. (1989b). Respiratory patterns associated with swallowing: Part 2. Neurologically impaired dysphagic patients. *Age and Ageing*, *18*, 173–176.

Selley, W.G., Flack, F.C., Ellis, R.E., & Brooks, W.A. (1990b). The Exeter dysphagia assessment technique. *Dysphagia*, *4*, 227–235.

Shawker, T.H., Stone, M., & Sonies, B.C. (1984). Sonography of speech and swallow. In R.C. Saunders & M.C. Hill (Eds.), *Ultrasound Annual* (pp. 237–260). New York: Raven Press.

Smith, J., Wolkove, N., Colacone, A., & Kreisman, H. (1989). Coordination of eating, drinking, and breathing in adults. *Chest*, *96*, 578–582.

Sonies, B.C. (1991). Ultrasound imaging and swallowing. In B. Jones & M. Donner (Eds.), *Normal and abnormal swallowing: Imaging in diagnosis and therapy* (pp. 109–117). New York: Springer-Verlag.

Sonies, B.C., Parent, L., Morrish, K., & Baum, B. (1988). Durational aspects of the oral-pharyngeal phase of swallow in normal adults. *Dysphagia*, *3*, 1–10.

Sorin, R., McClean, M.D., Ezerzer, F., & Fishbein, B.M. (1987). Electroglottographic evaluation of the swallow. *Archives of Physical Medicine and Rehabilitation*, *68*, 232–235.

Splaingard, M.L., Hutchins, B., Sulton, L.D., & Chaundhuri, G. (1988). Aspiration in rehabilitation patients: Videofluoroscopy vs bedside clinical assessment. *Archives of Physical Medicine and Rehabilitation*, *69*, 637–640.

Tanaka, E., Palmer, J., & Siebens, A. (1986). Bipolar suction electrodes for pharyngeal electromyography. *Dysphagia*, *1*, 39–40.

Thumfart, W.F. (1988). Electrodiagnosis of laryngeal nerve disorders. *Ear, Nose, and Throat Journal*, *67*, 380–393.

Appendix 8–A

Videofluoroscopic Examination of Oropharyngeal Swallowing Function

Patient Name: _____ ID#_____ Age____

Date of Examination:_____ Tape #: _____ Pt #:_____

Examining Clinician:_____ Referring Source_____

Present Dx :

Pertinent history:

Results of oral/facial examination:

Results of test swallows (if appropriate):

Source: © 1996, Adrienne L. Perlman, PhD.

Volumes and viscosities presented during VFE:

Key: a = always present; i = inconsistently present
1 = trace; 2 = mild; 3 = moderate; 4 = severe
Identify (circle) the volumes that are problematic

	Volumes Presented	LIQUID Thin / Thick		PASTE	SOLID
ORAL STAGE					
Poor bolus control					
drooling	—	—	—	—	—
base of tongue spillover	—	—	—	—	—
Bolus preparation					
absent	—	—	—	—	—
prolonged (seconds)	—	—	—	—	—
Poor bolus formation	—	—	—	—	—
Poor mastication	—	—	—	—	—
Incomplete tongue-palate contact	—	—	—	—	—
Poor bolus transport	—	—	—	—	—
Tongue pumping	—	—	—	—	—
Tongue thrust	—	—	—	—	—
Serial swallowing	—	—	—	—	—
Oral residue					
left lateral sulcus	—	—	—	—	—
right lateral sulcus	—	—	—	—	—
anterior floor of mouth	—	—	—	—	—
tongue blade	—	—	—	—	—
palate	—	—	—	—	—
Nasal regurgitation	—	—	—	—	—
Tremor	—	—	—	—	—
Oral transit time (seconds)	—	—	—	—	—
Other observations:					
PHARYNGEAL STAGE					
Initiation of pharyngeal stage					
delayed (seconds)	—	—	—	—	—
spillover to valleculae	—	—	—	—	—
spillover to pyriforms	—	—	—	—	—
Pharyngeal residue					
diffuse	—	—	—	—	—
valleculae R__ L__	—	—	—	—	—

	Volumes Presented	LIQUID Thin / Thick		PASTE	SOLID
aryepiglottic folds	___	____	____	____	____
pyriform sinuses R__ L__	___	____	____	____	____
Reduced velar elevation	___	____	____	____	____
Reduced hyoid displacement	___	____	____	____	____
Reduced laryngeal displacement	___	____	____	____	____
Reduced tongue base retraction	___	____	____	____	____
Deviant epiglottic function					
no inversion	___	____	____	____	____
partial inversion	___	____	____	____	____
prolonged inversion	___	____	____	____	____
BOT approximates epiglottis	___	____	____	____	____
C-shaped epiglottic curl	___	____	____	____	____
Impaired UES opening	___	____	____	____	____
Laryngeal penetration	___	____	____	____	____
before swallow	___	____	____	____	____
during swallow	___	____	____	____	____
after swallow	___	____	____	____	____
Aspiration					
before swallow	___	____	____	____	____
during swallow	___	____	____	____	____
after swallow	___	____	____	____	____
Impaired laryngeal closure	___	____	____	____	____
Asymmetrical level of folds	___	____	____	____	____
Pharyngeal transit time (sec)	___	____	____	____	____

Other observations:

CERVICAL ESOPHAGEAL STAGE

Retrograde flow	___	____	____	____	____
Upper esophageal sphincter residue	___	____	____	____	____
Diverticulum		____	____	____	____
Spasm/stricture		____	____	____	____
Fistula		____	____	____	____

Other observations:

RECOMMENDATIONS

Diet: NPO_____ PPO_____ Bolus size_____ Bolus viscosity_____
Follow solids with liquids_____ Other_____

Positioning: Chin tuck_____ Body position_____
  Turn head to: R___ L___ Tilt head to: R___ L___ Other_____

Maneuvers: Multiple swallows_____ Safe swallow_____
  Mendelsohn_____ Other_____

Exercises: Glottal closure _____ Pharyngeal constrictor _____
  Thermal-tactile stimulation _____ Chewing_____ Other_____

Referrals: Otolaryngology___ GI___ Neurology___ Prosthodontics___
  Dentistry___ Other_____

Appendix 8–B

FEES^{SM} Examination and Protocol

Patient Name: _____ ID#_____ Age_____
Date of Examination:_____ Tape #: _____ Pt #:_____
Examining Clinician:_____ Referring Source_____

I. **VELOPHARYNGEAL CLOSURE**
    At juncture of velum and nasopharynx, view sphincteric closure as the patient swallows and phonates nasal and non-nasal sounds and sentences. You may wish to return to the nasopharynx if nasal reflux is to be assessed.

II. **APPEARANCE OF HYPOPHARYNX AT REST**
    Scan around entire hypopharynx noting appearance and symmetry.

III. **BASE OF TONGUE RANGE/SYMMETRY**
    Task: Say "kuh-kuh-kuh" several times.
    Observe the extent of movement and symmetry.

IV. **RESPIRATION (ABDUCTION)**
    Observe laryngeal structures for rest breathing.
    Task: Sniff (note abduction).

V. **AIRWAY PROTECTION (ADDUCTION)**
    Task: Cough.

    Task: Hold your breath—at level of throat.

    Task: Hold your breath very tightly.

    Task: Hold your breath to the count of 7.

VI. **PHONATION (ABDUCTION/ADDUCTION)**
    Task: Hold "ee."

    Task: Repeat "hee-hee-hee" 5–7 times.

    Task: Count from 1–10.

    Task: Hold "ee" to the count of 7.

Source: Adapted from Susan Langmore, PhD. © 1996. FEES^{SM} is a service mark of Susan Langmore, PhD.

VII. PHARYNGEAL MUSCULATURE

Task: Hold your breath and blow out your cheeks as forcefully as possible.
Observe the depth and symmetry of pyriform sinuses.

Task: Strain your voice and say "ee" in a very loud, high voice.
Observe middle and inferior constrictors and estimate the extent and symmetry of contraction.

VIII. SWALLOWING SECRETIONS/SALIVA

Place two drops of food coloring on tongue.
Observe amount and location of secretions in lateral channels, in laryngeal vestibule, and/or subglottally.

Note: If secretions are seen at the glottis immediately on insertion of the endoscope, withhold green food coloring until after ice chips are given.

IX.   SWALLOWING FOOD AND LIQUID

All foods and liquids are colored with green food coloring.
Guidelines for standard examination:
- Increase the amount with each presentation unless aspiration occurs.
- Repeat any amount that results in aspiration, unless the aspiration is severe.
- Discontinue that amount if aspiration occurs twice.
- Try less than 5 cc only if patient at high risk for aspiration.
- The order of consistencies will vary, depending upon the patient's needs.
- Try therapeutic maneuvers at all appropriate points during the exam (e.g., head turn, chin tuck, effortful swallow, hold breath-swallow sequence, supraglottic swallow, Mendelsohn maneuver, dry swallows).
- Modify the exam and the instructions, as the situation warrants.

A. *Ice chips*
   Begin with this consistency if patient is NPO at present and/or appears to be at high risk for aspiration.
   Task: Swallow one ice chip. Repeat at least once.

B. *Pureed food*
   Task: Swallow (applesauce). Administer via syringe/spoon: 5cc, 10 cc, 15 cc.

C. *Soft solid food*
   Task: Chew and swallow (cheese sandwich.) Allow patient to take a bite-sized portion. Repeat for two "bites."

D. *Thin liquid*
   Task: Swallow milk (or other translucent liquid).
   Administer via syringe/straw as follows:

5 cc, 10 cc, 15 cc, 20 cc five consecutive sips from straw.
E. *Thick liquid*
Optional task, if aspiration of thin liquids occurs:
Task: Swallow (milkshake) or other translucent material.
Administer via syringe/straw:
5 cc, 10 cc, 15 cc, 20 cc five consecutive sips from straw.

X.   LARYNGOPHARYNGEAL SENSATION
Reduced sensation is suspected if the patient has shown reduced reaction to the presence of the scope or reduced awareness of residue, penetration, or aspiration.

Scoring a FEES exam: abnormal findings

A.   **Part I: Scoring hypopharyngeal/laryngeal function for airway protection, respiration, phonation, and sensation.**
• Reduced velopharyngal closure for phonation.
• Altered/abnormal anatomy that could impair swallowing (e.g., edema, asymmetry, shallow lateral channels, no vallecular space, the effects of head and neck surgery, etc.).
• Weak, reduced tongue movement; reduced pharyngeal constrictor movement; reduced laryngeal (arytenoid, true vocal-fold) movement.
• Inability of larynx to protect the airway for breath-holding, coughing, throat-clearing, phonation (adduction): "Laryngeal incompetence."
• Irregular, fast rate of respiratory cycles.
• Inability of larynx to sustain breath-holding.
• Reduced frequency of spontaneous swallow (3–5 minutes).
• Excess secretions:
    0 = No excess.
    1 = Excess in valleculae and/or pyriforms.
    2 = Excess in laryngeal vestibule or being aspirated.
• Lack of patient response to excess secretions.

B.   **Part II: Scoring swallowing function, efficacy of therapeutic maneuvers.**
• Velopharyngeal incompetence (viewed from the nasopharynx):
    Incomplete closure observed during the swallow; observed in speech during phonation of nonnasal phonemes
    Nasal reflux observed?

- Spillage into hypopharynx before initiating swallow:
  During oral preparation or attempt to initiate swallow?
  Time (in ms) that bolus is in view before white-out (more than 1
    second?)
  Location of bolus head as white-out begins (lower than valleculae?)
  Did the bolus spill over into the laryngeal vestibule?
  What was the point of entry?
- Status of laryngeal closure before and at onset of swallow:
  If spillage has occurred, were true vocal cords adducted during spill-
    age?
- Reduced laryngeal elevation, inferred from retroversion of epiglottis
    and associated with hyoid elevation; visual indication of laryngeal
    elevation
- Weak swallow with incomplete white-out. Lasted less than 650 ms?
- Excess residue after the swallow:
  Location and amount of residue.
  Did the patient spontaneously dry swallow to clear the residue?
  How many dry swallows did the patient perform spontaneously?
  Did the patient need to be cued to dry swallow?
  Were the dry swallows effective in clearing the residue?
    How many were needed?
  Was there build-up of residue over several new bolus presentations?
  Did the residue eventually penetrate the laryngeal vestibule? When?
    Was it aspirated?
- Laryngeal penetration:
  Point of entry? (anterior, lateral, posterior into vestibule)
  When did penetration occur? (before, during, after swallow)
- Aspiration:
  When did it occur? (before, during, after the swallow)
  Phase in respiration cycle (estimate from laryngeal adduction/abduc-
    tion)
  Patient response to aspiration; effectiveness of response (i.e., did it
    clear the bolus?)
- Was fatigue noted during the exam? How did it affect the swallow?
- Hypoasthesia/reduced sensation:
  Awareness of patient to residue, aspiration.
  Directly assess by *lightly* toughing base of tongue, posterior pharyngeal
    walls, tip of epiglottis.

Appendix 8–C

Ultrasound Examination of Swallowing

Patient Name: _____ **ID#**_____ **Age**_____
Date of Examination:_____ **Tape #:** _____ **Pt #:**_____
Examining Clinician:_____ **Referring Source**_____

I.   PLACEMENT OF TRANSDUCER
A. Begin with the sagittal or midline view (S) by placing the transducer in the soft area behind the center of the mandible.
B. Move the transducer to the left or right to get the best view of the curved surface of the tongue.
C. Rotate transducer back until hyoid shadow appears.
D. Leave the tranducer in this spot so you can track the motion of the hyoid.
E. Give the command to swallow and observe the sequence without saliva. Repeat this three times.
F. Give water, or any liquid, and repeat command.
G. Rotate transducer 90° at midline (in either direction) to obtain the coronal (C) view.

II.   ANATOMIC LANDMARKS seen on sagittal view (S) and coronal view (C).
A. Tongue surface midline (C & S) ____
B. Central groove on coronal view (C) ____
C. Genioglossus muscle (C & S) _____
D. Floor muscles (C & S) _____
E. Palate (C & S)—not always visible _____
F. Hyoid (S) and mandible (C & S) shadows _____
G. Muscle attachments at hyoid (S) _____
H. Pharynx—(S only) _____
I. Vallecula shadow, upper border of epiglottis _____

III.   MEASUREMENT OF THE DURATION OF SWALLOWING
A. Made from sagittal view from movement of hyoid bone.
B. Measurements should be done from stop–frame-by-frame analysis with the video editor. Measurement begins at the frame when hyoid bone begins to move forward/upward.

Source: © 1996, Barbara C. Sonies, PhD.

C. The measurement at the end of the swallow is the frame when the hyoid returns to resting position.

D. The total time is then measured by subtracting the starting time from the ending time. Time at end of movement minus time of initial movement of hyoid bone = total time of swallowing event.

IV. SWALLOWING ABNORMALITIES SEEN ON ULTRASOUND

A. Some patients are delayed in initiation of a swallow; this needs to be mentioned in the description of their swallows.

B. Some patients need several preparatory gestures to swallow; this is included in the total time.

C. Some patients have a forward/upward motion of the hyoid and others hold the hyoid forward for longer than expected or need multiple swallows to transport a bolus. The total time includes these abnormal components.

D. Swallowing observations from ultrasound:
   — Slow, irregular, or jerking motions of hyoid and tongue.
   — Density changes in the tongue muscles.
   — Fat deposits in the tongue muscles.
   — Asymmetry of floor muscles during bolus transport.
   — Asymmetry of tongue during bolus transport or resting.
   — Tongue pumping.
   — Tongue rigidity or spasms.
   — Mid-tongue blade dipping patterns.
   — Lingual dystonia.
   — Gestures that do not result in a swallow.
   — Pooling of secretions in oropharynx.
   — Chug/swallow. _____
   — Abnormal chewing or bolus lateralization patterns. _____
   — Multiple swallows for small bolus. _____
   — Any audible swallowing sounds. _____

V. BIOFEEDBACK FOR SWALLOWING THERAPY

A. Tracking bolus transport.
B. Tracking and imitation of proper temporal sequences.
C. Feedback on safe (supraglottic) swallow technique.
D. Feedback on Mendelsohn maneuver.
E. Feedback on tongue/hyoid activity.

CHAPTER 9

Instrumental Imaging Technologies and Procedures

Kenneth L. Watkin and Jeri L. Miller

Today, the dysphagia specialist has the unique opportunity to access a variety of technologies and instrumental procedures from which to assess and treat the individual with a swallowing disorder. Clinicians are challenged because they must know the purpose and function of each method to assess characteristics of swallowing dysfunction and provide objective information to guide in clinical decisions for treatment interventions. The clinician must be aware of the advantages and limitations of each technology and its cost, benefits, and ultimate impact on the patient. The use of many new technologies requires familiarity with a variety of procedures across many disciplines including radiology, otolaryngology, nuclear medicine, and gastroenterology. Knowledge of the instrumental procedure that best addresses the management of the presenting dysphagic condition is thus a combined cooperative effort of both diagnostician and therapist. What are the criteria from which to choose a specific technique? What are the benefits of one technique versus another and, most importantly, can a particular technology address the presenting clinical problem and provide the necessary information to ensure efficacious treatment?

This chapter will briefly review several imaging technologies currently available for use in the diagnosis and treatment of dysphagia. The general purpose and design of each technology will be described along with its limitations and advantages. In addition, new imaging methods currently being developed for clinical and research applications will be introduced to familiarize the reader with emerging instrumental approaches designed to enhance our understanding of normal and disordered swallowing processes. The goal of this chapter is to provide the dysphagia clinician with basic information that can assist in the selection of an appropriate instrumental procedure and provide new perspectives on technological approaches for the assessment and treatment of dysphagia. Because the authors' interests focus on the research and development of applications of ultrasound technologies, new state-of-the-art techniques and current trends in technologic developments will be emphasized in the final section.

INSTRUMENTAL IMAGING TECHNOLOGIES

The most familiar technologies used in dysphagia evaluation have provided static or dynamic images of the anatomy and physiology of swallowing. These technologies vary in how they acquire and display visual information. The most common methods include radiographic, magnetic resonance, ultrasound, and fiberoptic imaging. Each procedure has its own advantages and limitations, and addresses a specific aspect of the swallowing process.

Radiographic Imaging

Videofluorography

Radiographic imaging is the most common and accepted form of visual imaging in dysphagia evaluation. X-ray videofluoroscopy (VFS) is recognized as the "gold standard" for visualizing both the anatomy and physiology of the swallowing mechanism and has made this modality the procedure most widely used by dysphagia specialists today. The pioneering work by Logemann (1983) and others (Dodds, Logemann, & Stewart, 1990; Donner, 1986; Ekberg & Nylander, 1982) have documented its validity and reliability as both a diagnostic and a clinical treatment tool. The purpose of VFS is to study the anatomy and physiology of the oral preparatory, oral, pharyngeal, and cervical esophageal stages of deglutition and to define management and treatment interventions to assist the patient to swallow both efficiently and safely (Logemann, 1983, 1993). Moreover, this technology was the fundamental method for continued research in understanding normal and abnormal swallowing processes and documenting the efficacy of many current treatment programs. (The application of this method was described in greater detail in Chapter 8).

Fluoroscopy is based upon the emission of photoelectric energy from a high-voltage source. The main instrumentation used is the fluoroscopy unit, which, when energized, produces X-rays to pass through the desired region. Differences in the absorption properties among different tissues produce the pattern that forms the radiographic image. This image is converted and displayed on a viewing monitor or recorded on videotape. On-line dynamic images of the swallow from regions extending from the lips to the cervical esophagus are easily distinguished. Video sampling of swallowing behaviors integrated with video counters or computer-based analysis packages provides a record of the timing and coordination of various structures throughout the swallow. Variables such as bolus size and texture (viscosity), head postures and positioning, or responses to swallowing maneuvers can be assessed directly to document appropriate intervention strategies. The presence or absence of laryngotracheal aspiration and the underlying etiology of the swallowing disorder are key reasons for using this imaging modality. In addition, the primary advantages of videofluorography are the capability to observe the activity of the bolus sagittally and antero-posteriorly during the entire swallowing event, and the ability to record and analyze, frame by frame, the actions of the bolus integrated with anatomical structures such as the tongue, velum, posterior pharyngeal wall, larynx, cricopharyngeous, and esophagus.

Newer applications of videofluoroscopy have been to acquire simultaneous and quantitative information regarding temporal and biomechanical measures of swallowing. These new applications require the use of an integrated computerized database with software analysis programs (e.g., Logemann, Kahrilas, Begelman, Dodds, & Pauloski, 1989; Potratz, Dengel, Robbins, & Brooks, 1993). Other new procedures have combined videofluorography with manometric recordings of pharyngeal pressure (Cerenko, McConnel, & Jackson, 1989) or electromyographic recordings of various muscle responses during swallowing (Logemann, 1993). These combined techniques provide methods to both visualize and quantify specific characteristics of the swallowing process.

The disadvantages of this technology are that without the use of radio-opaque contrast material, it is difficult to visualize soft tissue structures such as the vocal cords or muscles of the tongue and oropharynx. These structures can be obscured by the dentition or oropharyngeal cartilages. Foodstuffs are given in controlled amounts and must be coated with barium. All assessments require the use of a radiographic imaging suite, which can make access to the procedure difficult in certain settings or patient populations. In addition, videofluorography does not quantify the relative degree of aspirated material. Finally, although ionizing radiation levels are carefully considered during examinations, exposure constitutes a health risk, particularly in pediatric patients.

Computer Assisted Tomography

Computer tomography (CT) also uses radiographic imaging methods to visualize the anatomic structures of swallowing. Images are obtained and displayed as a result of differences in the electron density among soft tissue, fat, air, and bone. Cross-sectional images can provide information on the shape and area of the pharyngeal cavity from the glossopalatal junction to the upper esophageal sphincter. As with X-ray, CT best depicts calcified tissues; but, because of its increased sensitivity, CT can display more distinct details and finer discriminations between fatty and nonfatty tissues. This has made the technique invaluable for identifying lesions and various pathologies contributing to dysphagia. Its foremost use, therefore, is to distinguish anatomic structures and identify pathologic conditions. This form of instrumentation requires more sophisticated radiographic technologies and the expertise of a neurologist and/or radiologist. Its primary limitation is the inability to dynamically display movements of structures during swallowing.

Research efforts have been made to increase the CT image capture rate by using ultrafast scanners. These new developments have been reported to provide images of the horizontal plane of the oropharynx at rates of 17 frames/sec (Ergun, Kahrilas, Lin, Logemann, & Harig, 1993; Ergun, 1994). Ultrafast CT is considered relatively noninvasive and exposes the patient to less radiation than videofluoroscopy. Further applications of this technique may permit more rapid sequencing of CT images to derive information on the influence of bolus conditions on pharyngeal volumes and swallowing biomechanics.

Scintigraphy

Another radiographic technology used in the assessment of swallowing processes is scintigraphy. A small amount of radioactive material (e.g., ciTechnetium sulfur colloid) is mixed into normal foodstuffs. This radioisotope material allows the bolus to be detected and "labelled" by a specialized gamma scintillation camera. During the evaluation, the patient is seated upright in front of this camera at a slight oblique angle. The radiation emitted by the swallowed bolus is then imaged and measured as it flows throughout the aerodigestive tract. The scintigraphic images can be reviewed throughout the swallowing process to identify the presence of the bolus in the pharynx, lungs, or esophagus; this permits measurement of both the magnitude and timing of bolus movement. Applications of scintigraphic technology to functional analyses of swallowing have been reported by various researchers (e.g., Fisher & Malmud, 1986; Muz, Mathog, Miller, Rosen, & Borreo, 1987; Silver & van Nostrand, 1991, 1994). Scintigraphy's primary advantage is that it detects and quantifies aspiration; however, it cannot define the etiology of the aspirate nor identify the anatomy and swallowing physiology that may have contributed to its occurrence. Although not all facilities have this technology and the necessary technical support readily available, it provides an excellent means for assessing and quantifying subtracheal aspiration, reflux, and gastric motility. Other limitations include difficulties in accurately detecting laryngotracheal retention and the occurrence of false positive findings (Silver & van Nostrand, 1994).

New Radiographic Techniques: X-Ray Microbeam Evaluations

One newer application of radiographic technologies has been the use of X-ray microbeams to monitor displacements and temporal movements of oral-facial structures during swallowing. The instrumentation has been applied primarily in investigations of movements of the tongue and responses to bolus volumes during swallowing (Hamlet, 1989; Stone & Shawker, 1986). Other possible applications are the integration and coordination of movements of the tongue, lips, and jaw during mastication and bolus preparation (Ostry, Flanagan, Feldman, & Munhall, 1991). The tracking of structural movements is accomplished through the use of a high-energy, 1-mm diameter, electron beam, which is capable of detecting and recording rapid motions of small gold pellets affixed to various surface areas in a small region of interest. A special scintillation counter detects the strength of the beam along with the scanning direction to identify the position and timing of each pellet's movements. Only controlled amounts of radiation are required, and integration with advanced automated computer processing allows data to be rapidly collected for analysis. An advantage of this system is the ability to gather large amounts of data from multiple points during rapid movements. Exposure to radiation levels is less than that experienced during a routine dental examination (Hamlet, 1989). This technology's main limitation is that it cannot provide an on-line visual display of the movements of the structure. However, when combined with imaging techniques such as ultrasound, temporal-spatial data can be displayed with visual information to provide objective measures of swallowing. In addition, to obtain data from only a select number of reference points where radio-opaque pellets have been placed (e.g., the surface of the apex, blade, and dorsum of the tongue), X-ray microbeam examinations require the patient's cooperation. The system was developed primarily for research and, therefore, is not accessible, nor cost-effective, for nationwide patient evaluation. However, the results of studies using this technique could provide important baseline information that could aid in developing models of the integrations of the many structures involved in swallowing and that could be compared to data from other types of newer three-dimensional imaging technologies.

Non-Radiographic Imaging

Three major technologies for the visualization of swallowing that are based upon non-radiation sources are available: magnetic resonance imaging (MRI), ultrasound, and fiberoptics. As in radiographic imaging, each technology should be selected to provide information to address a specific presenting problem. Each technique has both limitations and advantages, which will be highlighted.

Magnetic Resonance Imaging

MRI uses alternating magnetic fields to create movements within molecules. Differences in the movements and amounts of these molecules within different structures are detected by magnetic sensors and displayed as an image. The technique provides greater detailing of soft tissues such as muscle, cartilage, surface mucosa, and vascular structures. Its resulting superior contrast resolution has made this form of imaging the technology of choice for identifying normal and abnormal structures within the oropharynx (Lufkin, Wortham, Dietrich, Hoover,

Larsson, Kangarloo, & Hanafee, 1986; Christianson, Lufkin, Vinuela, & Hanafee, 1987; Kassel, Keller, & Kuchorczyk, 1989). Other advantages of this technology are the ability to obtain multiplanar images of gross anatomic anatomy, fewer image artifacts from dental appliances, and the lack of exposure to ionizing radiation. The major disadvantages of the method are the time and expense to obtain the scan, the need for the patient to be in a supine position, and the requirement that the patient remain enclosed and motionless for long periods during the scanning sequence. Although recent instruments now enable images to be obtained more rapidly, the technology does not permit dynamic or repeated visualizations of swallowing.

Recent MRI research has taken advantage of its capability to finely detect soft-tissue structures in an effort to better understand the underlying anatomic structures involved in swallowing. Analyses of changes to muscular structure and function have provided clues regarding the pathophysiology of aging (DePaul & Engelhardt, 1991) and disease (Kim, Buchholz, Kumar, Donner, & Rosenbaum, 1987) in structures such as the tongue. Advanced image analysis techniques have great potential, especially when linked with newer image analysis technologies to provide important temporal and spatial quantitative information on the morphology of the oropharyngeal structures in persons with dysphagia. Future research efforts will thus combine MRI scanning with the application of algorithms and computerized analyses, which show promise to assist in the differential diagnostic process relative to neurologic conditions.

Fiberoptics

Using fiberoptics as an imaging tool in the study of swallowing has provided a means to obtain real-time visualizations of actual anatomic structures. Unlike other imaging techniques, fiberoptics presents a true color, three-dimensional anatomic view of portions of the pharynx and larynx through a flexible fiberoptic endoscope. This endoscope is reasonably small (3.5 mm) and, therefore, can be introduced transnasally or orally for viewing laryngopharyngeal structures extending from the velum to the vocal folds. Several studies (Bastian, 1991; Langmore, Schatz, & Olson, 1988) have demonstrated that this technology can provide information regarding airway protection and vocal-cord status, management of secretions, coordination of breath-holding and swallowing maneuvers, and laryngeal/pharyngeal sensitivity. Information regarding bolus transport before the swallow, particularly at the tongue dorsum-oropharynx junction, can be observed across a variety of postures and actual foodstuffs. Video recordings provide dynamic records, which can be used as educational or biofeedback tools.

Unlike the technologies presented previously, the measurement precision of fiberoptic images is difficult because of depth-of-view distortion. Information regarding oral and esophageal structures and their coordinated actions cannot be assessed. During the actual moment of bolus transport into the oropharynx, the lower segments of the pharynx, larynx, and esophagus are obscured from view because of the descent of the epiglottis and contraction of the pharyngeal walls around the bolus. The transitions from oral, pharyngeal, and esophageal stages cannot be determined, nor can many of the coordinated interactions of swallowing structures be viewed. In addition, some patient populations may not easily tolerate insertion of the scope.

A new application of this technology has been to combine endoscopic imaging with simultaneous electromyographic or videofluorographic recordings. The use of combined procedures is important in the applications of technologies for the study of dysphagia. Considered alone, each of the technologies described previously makes an important contribution to the understanding of the dynamics of swallowing but is not in-and-of-itself complete. The state-of-the-art is to provide both visual and quantifiable data through the integrated use of several technologies. This important next step must be taken to ensure that objective information is obtained to verify the effectiveness of our diagnostic and intervention strategies.

Ultrasound

Ultrasound imaging technology remains one of the safest and noninvasive means to evaluate specific aspects of swallowing. It is an important technology that has been applied to the study of the tongue and pharynx through the pioneering efforts of Shawker, Sonies, and colleagues (Shawker, Stone, & Sonies, 1984; Shawker, Sonies, Hall, & Baum, 1984; Shawker, Sonies, Stone, & Baum, 1984). Their germinal studies demonstrated that the technique could be used to visualize movements of the tongue, floor of the mouth, hyoid, and larynx during swallowing. The soft tissues of these structures are easily distinguished from the bolus, thus requiring no use of contrast material. Multiple planes of view can be obtained during swallowing of normal food boluses in everyday feeding situations, and across a variety of postures and swallowing maneuvers. Quantitative data regarding the timing and duration of lingual and bolus movements (Sonies, Parent, Morrish, & Baum, 1988; Stone & Shawker, 1986) have been derived from both normal and abnormal adults (Hamlet, Stone, & Shawker, 1988; Sonies, Ekman, Andersson, Adamson, Kaler, Markello, & Gahl, 1990), the elderly (Sonies, Stone, & Shawker, 1984), and infants (Weber, Woolridge, & Baum, 1986; Smith, Erenberg, Nowak, & Franken, 1985). Its safety and ease of use have made ultrasound a part of routine clinical examinations for oral and neck masses (Ishikawa, Ishii, Ono, Makimoto, Yamamoto, and Torizuka, 1983) and in the evaluation of pediatric patients (Kenny, Casas, & McPherson, 1989; Casas, Kenny, & McPherson, 1994).

The primary advantages of ultrasound are its safety and ease of use, and the ability to provide the dysphagia specialist with dynamic real-time data that can be collected repeatedly across a variety of bolus types and conditions. Moreover, ultrasound can be repeated easily and quickly. Thus, it can effectively assess clinical treatment efficacy over time and provide necessary objective documentation of behavioral changes of the swallow. Diagnostic ultrasound provides dynamic images, which can be stored on videotape for review and measurement. In addition, new applications are being developed to provide imaging of several regions of the oropharynx, including the oral cavity, pharynx, or laryngeal regions. These new applications are described in greater detail in the following text.

The disadvantage of ultrasound is that only soft-tissue structures are readily identifiable. Bone does not allow transmission of the sound wave, thus producing an echo-free or shadowed region within the image. The field of view is currently limited by the size of the transducer aperture used to obtain the image. Thus, the extent of the sonographic image is confined to a region extending from the anterior oral cavity to the posterior aspect of the hyoid bone. The tongue tip and hypopharynx are not always visible in adult subjects, nor can simultaneous views of laryngopharyngeal relationships be obtained.

High-frequency ultrasound probes (5–10 MHz), which were recently developed, now provide the resolution needed to obtain clear images of the tongue and its surrounding musculature (see Figure 9–1). This detailed resolution has provided a means to better detect oral soft-tissue masses. Image processing techniques such as colorization or contrast enhancement now allow the sonographer to identify more clearly both normal and abnormal tissue states. More recent research indicates that ultrasound may be used to analyze the pathophysiology of soft tissues of the oropharyngeal region. Although ultrasound cannot detect aspiration, recent research on contrast agents indicates that methods to better identify and quantify bolus transit may be developed (Kenny, D.J., 1995, personal communication). Finally, integration of ultrasound with high-speed data acquisition and three-dimensional software programs have provided methods from which a simple two-dimensional ultrasound recording can be displayed in three dimensions and objective data can be obtained regarding swallowing movements, bolus influences, and responses to treatment techniques (Cordaro, Stone, Goldstein, & Unser, 1991; Wang & Sonies, 1995; Wein, Böckler, & Klajman, 1991).

NEW APPROACHES TO THE USE OF ULTRASOUND TECHNOLOGY

The potential of future imaging technologies to provide the dysphagia therapist with greater detail of swallowing anatomy and multiple methods from which to describe and quantitate swallowing physiology is exciting. This section will provide examples of future trends in the field as demonstrated through our ongoing efforts in ultrasound technologies. Ultrasound has the potential to play a greater role in both the assessment and intervention of dysphagia. Because ultrasound can be used repeatedly, it provides an ideal visualization technique within the clinical setting and, when used in conjunction with other visualization methods, provides

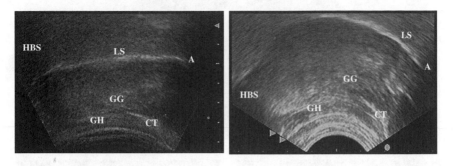

5 MHz probe   7.5 MHz probe

Figure 9–1 Comparison of ultrasound image quality. Echo signals from a 5 MHz and a 7.5 MHz ultrasound probe imaging the same adult tongue. The corresponding abbreviations are used for landmarks (LS: lingual surface; GG: genioglossus; GH: geniohyoid; HBS: hyoid bone shadow; CT: connective tissue; A: region near the lingual apex).

the clinician with the breadth of information needed for clinical application. Several new advances in the applications of ultrasound using computers for image acquisition, image processing, and image display have the potential to provide additional information for the practitioner.

Real-Time Assessment of Lateral Pharyngeal Wall Motion During Swallowing

Early work by Kelsey and his group at the University of Wisconsin in the late 1960s (e.g., Kelsey, Hixon, & Minifie, 1969) attempted to monitor the movements of the lateral pharynx. The movements of the pharynx are recognized to be important for the propulsion and clearance of the bolus during swallowing; however, its analysis has been primarily of the posterior pharyngeal wall during lateral videofluorographic imaging. Recently, Watkin and Miller (1996a, 1996b) have used multi-crystal, curved array, B-mode ultrasound systems to explore the potential of this method's application to the study of oropharyngeal swallowing.

An ultrasound transducer is placed along one side of the patient's neck to provide an image of the pharyngeal wall extending from the superior to mid-pharynx. The patient may be seated in a variety of postures, and any variety of bolus types can be used. Figure 9–2 presents examples of several different types of swallowing maneuvers analyzed using simultaneous recordings of B-mode ultrasound images along with the M-mode (time-motion mode) information. This simultaneous recording method provides a visual display of the actual movements of the

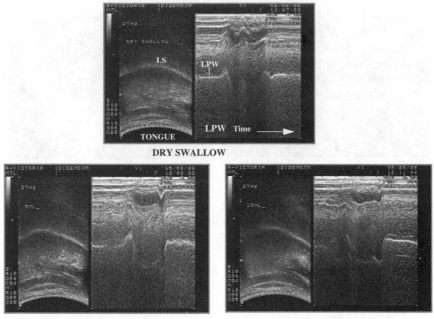

DRY SWALLOW

5 mL BOLUS SWALLOW   **10 mL BOLUS SWALLOW**

Figure 9–2 Lateral pharyngeal wall motion. Motion of the lateral pharyngeal wall (LPW) is presented for three different swallowing maneuvers: dry swallow; 5 mL bolus swallow; and 10 mL bolus swallow. The left half of each image contains the position of the tongue and the lingual surface (LS), and the right half contains the images of the LPW. Baseline is indicated in the middle of the image.

lateral wall and an on-line recording of the movements of selected regions. As can be seen, there are distinct differences in the on-line recording responses during differing swallow conditions. The timing of the bolus clearance can be determined easily by using the cursor measurement system available in all ultrasound machines. These preliminary data suggest that repeated observations of the lateral walls of the pharynx can be recorded. Moreover, it is conceivable that with the availability of small, portable, ultrasound machines the clinician could conduct a preliminary evaluation of oral and oropharyngeal swallowing behaviors at the bedside before initiating in-depth videofluoroscopy examinations. In addition, the clinician could use ultrasound imaging to assist in the training of swallowing maneuvers, and provide instant and continuous feedback during intervention.

Hyoid Bone Movement During Swallowing

One of the principal mechanical determinants of upper esophageal sphincter opening is the movement of the hyoid bone. The upward and forward movement of the bone reconfigures the oropharynx for swallowing. Thus, the movements of the hyoid are important clinical indicators of the patient's swallowing behavior pattern. The movements of the hyoid may be observed and measured using either videofluoroscopy or two-dimensional ultrasound, and may be measured from recorded video samples. Two different methods of recording the movements of the hyoid bone with ultrasound have been reported: (1) frame-by-frame estimation of hyoid bone movement (Cordaro & Sonies, 1993) and (2) utilization of duplex Doppler spectral analysis (Sonies & Wang, 1994; Sonies, Wang, & Sapper, 1996). Cordaro and Sonies (1993) developed a method to extract the changes in position of hyoid bone during a swallowing sequence. Their method extracted hyoid bone position frame by frame from a videotape. This method was designed to increase the accuracy of identification of the hyoid bone in each video frame because the hyoid bone is not visible on a two-dimensional ultrasound image, only its shadow is visible. Verification of the method included simultaneous videofluorography and ultrasound of single swallowing sequences with synchronized computer-assisted time marking to facilitate data analysis. Separate image processing strategies were designed to extract the hyoid image from the videofluorographic images and ultrasound images because ultrasound does not image the hyoid bone as a structure. Hyoid bone trajectories were similar in shape for both modalities. Because the pattern of hyoid movement and overall extent and timing of hyoid bone motion were similar, Watkin and Miller (1996a and 1996b) decided to explore the possibility of displaying the real-time B-mode images projected along a time axis. This type of display is similar in concept to sound spectrographic displays. That is, the time axis is composed of individual B-mode images placed in a stack from left to right (X axis or time). Movement would be displayed in the Y axis. The intensity of the ultrasound image would be projected toward the viewer. Thus, like the sound spectrogram, the display is three-dimensional with time composed of a stack of images. This technique has the potential for visualization of both the antero-posterior movement of the hyoid shadow movement and the superior-inferior movement. Moreover, this would eliminate the need for time-consuming image processing. To explore this application of real-time ultrasound, two different types of swallowing patterns were recorded. Using a Macintosh PPC 7100/66 with a video frame grabber, the subject was seated upright with the ultrasound probe in the submandibular position; a region of interest window within the two-dimensional ultrasound image was set using a trackball; and a swallowing sequence was digitized at 27 frames per second and stored on the hard drive of the computer. Two subjects (one female, one male) each produced two independent swallow maneuvers: a normal 10 mL swallow of water and a 10 mL Mendelsohn maneuver swallow. Figures 9–3 and 9–4 present the normal and Mendelsohn swallowing data, respectively. Image acquisition time was brief (a few seconds) because only a single swallow was recorded, whereas image projection time was approximately 60 sec. The time-varying tracings of the swallowing patterns clearly differ. The antero-posterior and superior-inferior movements of the hyoid for the normal swallow seem to have a similar time course to those reported by Kahrilas and Logemann (1993). For comparative purposes, we digitally traced the hyoid movements in each direction and plotted them in a Cartesian coordinate system (see Figure 9–5). The trajectories are similar to those reported by Cordaro and Sonies (1993) and Kahrilas and Logemann (1993). This is another example of the possible application of ultrasound to assist in understanding the dynamics of the swallowing event, especially the major determinants of upper esophageal sphincter opening. The development of this technique underscores the need for the develop-

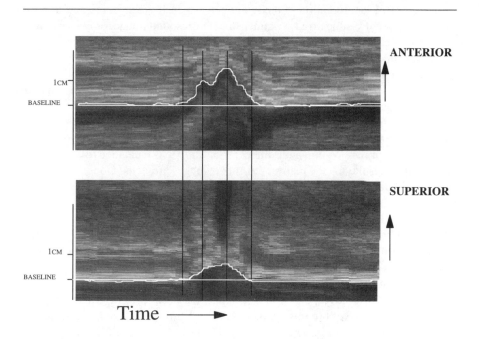

Figure 9–3 Time plot of hyoid bone movement for a normal adult male completing a 10 mL bolus swallow. The antero-posterior movement of the hyoid is presented in the upper half of the figure. In the lower half of the figure, the superior-inferior movement of the hyoid bone is presented. The movement of the hyoid bone is identified with a solid white line whereas the baseline is marked with a dashed line.

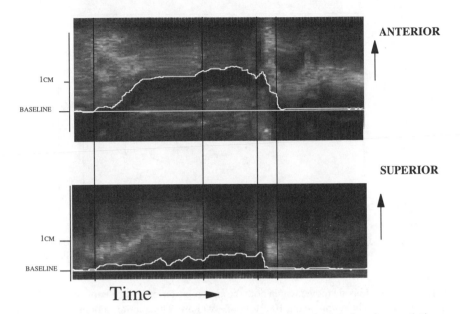

Figure 9–4 Time plot of hyoid bone movement for a normal adult female completing a 10 mL Mendelsohn bolus swallow. The antero-posterior movement of the hyoid is presented in the upper half of the figure. In the lower half of the figure, the superior-inferior movement of the hyoid bone is presented. The movement of the hyoid bone is identified with a solid white line whereas the baseline is marked with a dashed line.

---

ment of accurate, real-time image acquisition and display technologies, which will assist the clinician in evaluating their patients and verifying treatment outcomes.

Three-Dimensional Ultrasound

Ultrasonography of the oropharynx has been recognized as a safe imaging technique. One of the difficulties facing the clinician is evaluating the form and function of this musculature. The two-dimensional imaging techniques (i.e., videofluoroscopy and ultrasound) described previously provide views of single planes but are unable to visualize the anatomy in three dimensions. There have been several noteworthy attempts to assist in understanding the complex three-dimensional geometry of the aerodigestive tract. Watkin and Rubin (1989), Baer, Gore, Gracco, and Nye (1991), Cordaro et al. (1991), Lin, Chen, Kahrilas, and Hertz (1994), and Wang and Sonies (1995) all have used wireframe or surface approximations of the oropharynx. To understand the relationships between

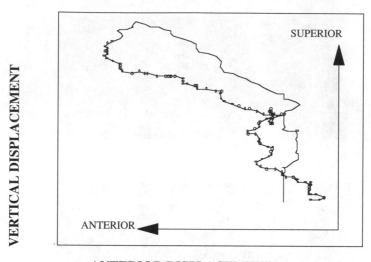

ANTERIOR DISPLACEMENT

Figure 9–5 Hyoid bone movement in both the antero-posterior and superior-inferior directions for a male who completed a 10 mL bolus swallow. This motion-motion plot depicts the upward and forward movement of the hyoid in the beginning of the swallow (open circles); the second phase continues upward but slightly posterior; whereas the final phase reveals a downward and backward movement. The second and third phases are presented as a solid line.

muscle groups, the effects of different contractile muscle states, and the effects of these muscles on the surfaces of the oropharynx, visualization of all the structural anatomy is required. Watkin (Watkin & Myre, 1989; Watkin, Nuwayhid, & Khalife, 1991; Watkin, Baer, Mathur, Jones, Hakim, Diout, Nuwayhid, & Khalife, 1993) has recently developed a research-quality, three-dimensional, ultrasonographic imaging technique that uses hardware and software techniques incorporated into a stand-alone workstation for use with existing ultrasound machines. Watkin's technique provides a reliable, valid, cost-effective, and safe means of acquiring three-dimensional images for clinical or research purposes (Cala, Watkin, Macklem, & Rochester, 1993; Kenyon, Cala, Watkin, Macklem, & Rochester, 1993; Gallagher, Watkin, & Plante, 1995).

Two methods are currently used to create three-dimensional ultrasonic images. One method involves a mechanical system to move the ultrasound transducer around a constant axis in fixed steps, record the images at each step, interpolate between the image slices, and display the reconstructed three-dimensional images. These mechanical scanning systems create pyramidally shaped three-dimensional images. Such systems have a limited number of slices that can be used to create a three-dimensional reconstruction, which degrades the resolution of the final image, reduces the accuracy of any calculation from such image data sets, and requires interpolation to provide a complete three-dimensional image. Because the sonographer must hold the mechanical scanner above the regions of interest, small movements of the sonographer's hand as well as subject movement add distortion to the resultant image. In addition, most mechanical scanning systems use a pyramidal image field, which reduces the size of the sampling region close to the transducer; this is problematic when babies or small children are being scanned. The second method involves the free movement of the ultrasound transducer and, therefore, requires localization of the position and orientation of the transducer while images are accumulated simultaneously (Watkin, Baer, Jones, Mathur, Hakim, Diout, Nuwayhid, & Khalife, 1993; Watkin, Mathur, Baer, Jones, Hakim, Diout, Nuwayhid, & Khalife, 1993). This method has several advantages over the mechanical method: it permits the acquisition of many closely spaced images, thereby reducing the need for extensive interpolation between slices during reconstruction; it increases image resolution in the lateral domain; and it permits the imaging of small muscles near the body surface.

The three-dimensional imaging system described here—freehand, rectangular, high-resolution, high-density, computer-enhanced, three-dimensional, ultrasound images (RHR-HD 3DUS)—was developed at McGill University (Watkin et al., 1993). This imaging method consists of three principal components: an ultrasound system, a localization device to track the position and orientation of the ultrasound transducer, and a computer to capture in real time the ultrasound images simultaneously with the localization records while the sonographer slowly moves the transducer across the abdomen above the fetal head/brain. These images are non-coplanar and need to be transformed into a series of parallel (co-planar) slices for three-dimensional visualization and measurement. The images and the localization data for each image are then transformed (reconstructed) into a series of images used to create a three-dimensional image using computer volume rendering techniques. This system is described in the following text.

Localizing the Probe

Critical to this system is the six-degree-of-freedom tracking device used to record the position and orientation of the transducer while it is moved from one end of the fetal brain to the other. The tracking system used is an AC-pulsed inductive magnetic coil transmitting/sensing system (Polhemus Navigation, Inc., Colchester, Vermont, *3Space Tracker*). An orthogonally wound transmitter emits low-level magnetic waves in the XYZ directions. A similarly wound, small sensor detects these magnetic waves. The values are used to determine the XYZ position of the sensor in global space as well as its orientation (pitch, roll, and yaw). Thus the sensor, when attached to an ultrasonic transducer (probe), sends data on the XYZ position of the transducer and the orientation of the transducer. These data are transmitted at 19,200 baud. The tracker has a resolution of +/– 1 mm, which is less than or equal to the lateral resolution of ultrasound systems (range: 1.0–4.0 mm). The tracker data are synchronized with the ultrasound images, which are simultaneously digitized using a video grabbing board which is also in the computer. Controlling software permits the selection of the rate of image acquisition. Ultrasound images and tracker data are captured at a rate the user can select (single-frame mode or 2–27 frames per second). This will result in an ensemble of 200–800 images depending upon the rate of movement of the transducer and the size of the scan region. Unlike the mechanical scanning methods, large or small regions may be imaged.

Acquiring and Reconstructing 3DUS Images

The RHR-HD 3DUS technique requires that the clinician move the probe slowly across the regions of interest. This permits the software and hardware to gather the many overlapping images used in the reconstruction process. This results in ensembles of overlapping images and most of the images are not parallel to each other. Creating a three-dimensional image from a nonparallel data set requires a resampling algorithm (Watkin et al., 1993). The resampling algorithm takes each of the pixels in each of the acquired two-dimensional images and its associated pixel location and orientation data and reconstructs all the pixels into a three-dimensional volume where the images are parallel to each other. The original two-dimensional images are processed at a rate of 1.2 Mpixels per second using a Silicon Graphics, Inc. Indigo workstation. The result is a series of parallel slices. The time needed for typical three-dimensional image reconstructions ranges from 45 to 120 seconds depending upon the image size, the number of images, and type of computer. Once the parallel slices have been created, the image may be visualized. The data are in the form of voxels and may be projected (visualized) using any commercially available volume rendering software. The voxel sizes of the images gathered vary with magnification and range from $0.02 \times 0.019 \times 0.1$ cm to $0.059 \times 0.058 \times 0.1$ cm. These volume pixel values are comparable in precision to those reported in MRI studies. Sample images of an in vivo adult tongue are presented in Figure 9–6. These images provide an example of the type of detail obtained using 3DUS reconstructions. A limited number of specific landmarks of lingual anatomy are identified to help the reader understand three-dimensional imaging of the tongue.

Image Segmentation and Volume Determination

The determination of regional volumes of three-dimensional ultrasound images of the tongue involves several steps: (1) the identification of landmarks that can be

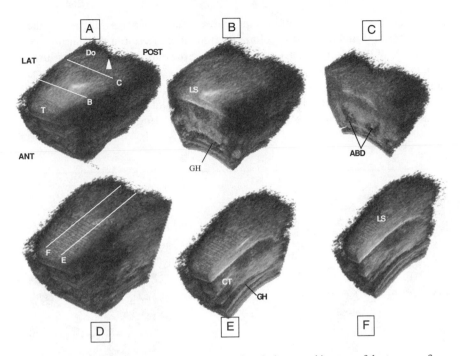

Figure 9–6 Three-dimensional volume rendered ultrasound images of the tongue of a normal adult male and associated landmarks. The anterior (ANT) and posterior (POST) parts of the image are identified along with a region near the tip of the tongue (T); the lingual surface (LS), the geniohyoid muscle (GH), the connective tissue (CT), the anterior belly of the digastric (ABD), the dorsal surface of the tongue (Do), and an arrowhead indicating the region of the tongue groove. Section A depicts the complete tongue in three dimensions. The lines B and C indicate the subsequent transverse slices through the tongue. Section D depicts the whole tongue with the sagittal slices indicated as the lines E and F. The corresponding slices are presented.

replicated in the resulting three-dimensional image, (2) computer-generated planes for the determination of regions of interest, (3) the identification of the edge of each region in each three-dimensional slice, and (4) the calculation of the volume of the region of interest. Watkin and Miller (1996b) have developed software based upon surface modelling techniques. This software uses the three-dimensional dataset created for volume visualization and permits the operator to place a "stretchable membrane" around an identified region in the three-dimensional images. This membrane can be stretched (deformed) to match the boundaries of the region within the image and the software instantaneously provides a calculation of the volume of the region. Figure 9–7 provides a sample image illustrating the software interface and associated volume regions identified in a normal in vivo adult tongue. Volume estimations calculated using the elastic deformable volume estimation software (Watkin & Miller, 1996b) were compared with estimations calculated using commercially available ultrasound machines (Figure 9–8). Using an 80 cc and 50 cc elliptical tissue mimicking phantom placed within a tissue equivalent medium errors of estimation of the volume using this volume estima-

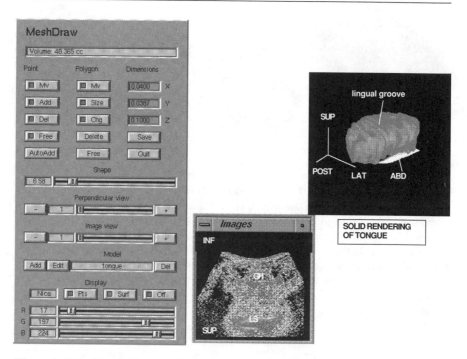

Figure 9–7 Surface rendering and volume measurement of the tongue. MeshDraw is a tool used to identify surfaces, internal muscular landmarks, and the associated volumes of these objects. The objects are projected as colored surfaces. The panel to the left contains all the control buttons needed for viewing and measurement. The panel marked "Images" contains a sample view of the tongue seen in Figure 9–6. The image is inverted with LS indicating the lingual surface and GH the geniohyoid. Inferior (INF) and superior (SUP) are marked. The last panel depicts the three-dimensional surface model of the tongue. The anterior belly of the digastric (ABD) can be seen below the tongue body. Superior (SUP), posterior (POST), and lateral (LAT) projection planes are indicated. The lingual groove is also evident.

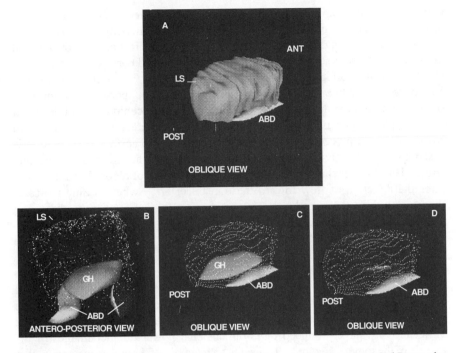

Figure 9–8 Surface rendering and volume measurement of the tongue. MeshDraw also includes the ability to convert surfaces to points thereby revealing structures below each surface. The tongue surface presented in Figure 9–7 is presented in section A. In section B the tongue has been rotated into an antero-posterior projection and the surface of the tongue (LS) converted to points. The relationship of the geniohyoid muscle (GH) to the two parts of the anterior belly of the digastric is revealed. In section C, the projection has been rotated to provide an oblique view where one of the ABD muscles cannot be seen because of the surface rendering of the GH. Section D is the same oblique view as C, except the surface rendering of the GH has been converted to points. Each surface object can be color-coded, and can be removed or added with a click of the mouse button.

---

tion software varied from 1.5–2.2%, whereas the estimations provided using the built-in volume estimations routines in the ultrasound machine varied from 1.5–4.5%.

Quantification of Echogenicity of the Tongue

Finally, new developments in ultrasound imaging techniques focus on extending their use beyond temporal and spatial measurements to objective quantification of the soft tissue structures that are the main features for sonographic imaging.

Ultrasound technologies promise, especially three-dimensional techniques, to provide information on the distribution of blood vessels in both the oral and pharyngeal cavities. Two different forms of ultrasound visualization can now be used to assist in detecting and measuring not only muscle and connective tissues, but also the vascularization of structures such as the tongue. This information is important for the study of swallowing, particularly regarding persons receiving tissue grafts, chemotherapy, or radiation therapies. This technique used traditional color doppler display of blood flows available on commercial machines and/or in advanced image processing power doppler programs. The former technique is based upon the power spectrum of the doppler shift determined by the ultrasound arrays. This doppler shift is color-coded by the direction of blood flows: red indicates the direction of flow toward the transducer array whereas blue indicates flows away from the transducer. Thus, during traditional gray-scale ultrasound imaging, the combined use of doppler imaging allows the detection and measurement of both venous and arterial blood flow. Miller and Watkin (1996b) have piloted this technique while analyzing the blood flow to the tongue and floor of the mouth during various muscular contractions and bolus swallows. Not only can blood flow be mapped, but differences can be observed during and after muscle contractions and in response to the swallow. An exciting possibility is to produce these images as three-dimensional color doppler displays. Recently, Watkin and Miller (1996b) have produced three-dimensional power doppler images of the vessels of the tongue. Figure 9–9 presents an example of three-dimensional power doppler. Figures 9–9A and 9–9B show the three-dimensional image as seen in Figure 9–6 whereas Figures 9–9C and 9–9D show the distribution of vessels (color-coded in red and displayed in this text as black) in the tongue from several different perspectives. This technique has potential for use in persons with dysphagia as a result of oral cancers to determine the viability of tissue grafts, the disruption of circulation due to the presence of tumors or damage from reconstructive surgery, or the recovery of function as a result of treatments and intervention.

A promising image processing technique is the quantitative analysis of the actual soft tissue regions within an ultrasound image field. Miller and Watkin (1996a) have described pilot data on the quantification of lingual musculature and connective tissue distributions using tissue characterization analyses of regional ultrasound intensity information. Figures 9–10 and 9–11 are samples of the echogenic characteristics of a normal subject (see Figure 9–10). A patient with a lingual myopathy (see Figure 9–11) can be seen to demonstrate different echogenic characteristics at rest, during light press, and during hard press of the tongue apex on the alveolar ridge. To quantify the echo intensity patterns, digital ultrasound images of the lingual structures are defined within specific polygonal regions, and the statistical properties of the intensity distributions of the tissues are analyzed. Differences in muscle force have been found to correlate with differ-

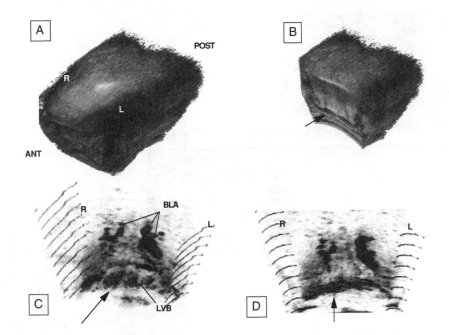

Figure 9–9 Three-dimensional volume rendered images of an adult tongue and the associated three-dimensional blood flow derived from three-dimensional color doppler reconstructions. Section A depicts the complete three-dimensional tongue whereas section B depicts the tongue sliced in the transverse plane. Sections C and D are different view projections of the blood flow patterns of the same tongue. The lines on the side are 1 cm calibration markers. Left (L) and right (R) are marked in the panels. BLA means branches of the lingual artery whereas LVB refers to the lingual vascular bed. The arrow indicates the region of the vascular bed in Sections B, C, and D.

ences in the image region intensity values. Thus, we have a new way to consider muscle physiology via a simple, repeatable, and noninvasive technology. The results have suggested that tissue characterization techniques may be useful in quantifying normal from abnormal pathologies, monitoring changes to the lingual musculature in response to treatment or therapy, or assessing changes to lingual structures in response to aging processes. The implications for both assessment and intervention of various approaches to the development of muscle force are clear. Although this application is in its early stages, it has great potential. In addition, this same technique can be applied to the three-dimensional images discussed previously and thereby could provide information on the regional distribution of force.

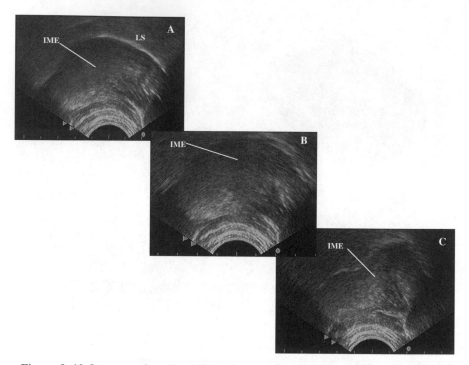

Figure 9–10 Intramuscular echogenicity changes with muscle contraction for a normal adult female. Section A (rest), B (light pressing of the tongue against the hard palate), and C (hard pressing against the palate) demonstrate the change in echogenicity in the region of intramuscle echogenicity (IME). The lingual surface is identified with LS.

CONCLUSION

Understanding the complex anatomic and physiologic biomechanics of swallowing has been elucidated by the advent of instrumental technologies. A variety of techniques from which to visualize and measure swallowing are now available to both the clinician and researcher. As we continue to expand the use of imaging technologies to detect and quantify swallowing disorders, the possibilities to increase both our knowledge and expertise in instrumentation remain challenging for those working in this field. Ultimately, many available imaging technologies ensure the accurate assessment and management plan for safe and efficient nutritional and hydrational intake in the variety of patients presenting with swallowing disorders.

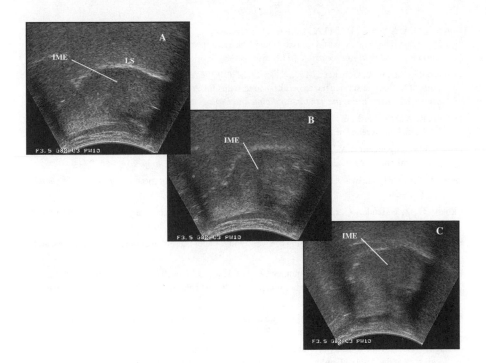

Figure 9–11 Intramuscular echogenicity changes with muscle contraction for an adult with dysphagia and neuromyopathy. Section A (rest), B (light pressing of the tongue against the hard palate), and C (hard pressing against the palate) demonstrate the change in echogenicity in the region IME. The lingual surface is identified with LS.

REFERENCES

Baer, T., Gore, J.C., Gracco, L.C., & Nye, P.W. (1991). Analysis of vocal tract shape using magnetic resonance imaging: Vowels. *Journal of the Acoustical Society of America*, *90*, 799–828.

Bastian, R.W. (1991). Videoendoscopic evaluation of patients with dysphagia: An adjunct to the modified barium swallow. *Otolaryngology—Head and Neck Surgery*, *104*, 339–350.

Cala, S.J., Watkin, K.L., Macklem, P.T., & Rochester, D.F. (1993). Ultrasonography of respiratory motion. *American Review of Respiratory Diseases*, *147*, A694.

Casas, M., Kenny, D., & McPherson, K. (1994). Swallowing ventilation interactions during oral swallow in normal children and children with cerebral palsy. *Dysphagia*, *9*, 40–46.

Cerenko, D., McConnel, F., & Jackson, R. (1989). Quantitative assessment of pharyngeal bolus driving forces. *Otolaryngology—Head and Neck Surgery*, *100*, 57–63.

Christianson, R., Lufkin, R.B., Vinuela, F., & Hanafee, W. (1987). Normal magnetic resonance imaging anatomy of the tongue, oropharynx, hypopharynx, and larynx. *Dysphagia*, *1*, 119–127.

194 DYSPHAGIA: A CONTINUUM OF CARE

Cordaro, M.A. & Sonies, B.C. (1993). An image processing scheme to quantitatively extract and validate hyoid bone motion based on real-time ultrasound recordings of swallowing. *IEEE Transactions on Biomedical Engineering, 40* (8), 841–844.

Cordaro, M., Stone, M., Goldstein, M.H., & Unser, M. (1991). A dynamic three-dimensional representation of the tongue surface based on ultrasound scans for time-varying localizations. *Annual Conference of the IEEE Engineering in Medicine and Biology Society, 13* (4), 1885–1886.

DePaul, R., & Engelhardt, E. (1991). Age related tongue tissue changes using MRI. Paper presented at the Annual Conference of the American Speech-Language and Hearing Association, Seattle, WA.

Dodds, W.J., Logemann, J.A., & Stewart, E.T. (1990). Radiological assessment of abnormal oral and pharyngeal phases of swallowing. *American Journal of Roentgenology, 154,* 965–974.

Donner, M. (1986). The evaluation of dysphagia by radiography & other methods of imaging. *Dysphagia, 1,* 49–50.

Ekberg, O., & Nylander, G. (1982). Cineradiography of the pharyngeal stage of deglutition in 150 individuals without dysphagia. *British Journal of Radiology, 55,* 252–257.

Ergun, G.A. (1994). Ultrafast CT imaging of swallowing. Paper presented at the Swallowing Research Symposium, Chicago, IL.

Ergun, G.A., Kahrilas, P.J., Lin, S., Logemann, J.A., & Harig, J.M. (1993). Shape, volume, and content of the deglutitive pharyngeal chamber imaged by ultrafast computerized technology. *Gastroenterology, 105,* 1396–1403.

Fisher, R., & Malmud, L. (1986). Scintigraphic techniques for the study of gastrointestinal motor function. *Advances in Internal Medicine, 31,* 395–418.

Gallagher, T.M., Watkin, K.L., & Plante, E.L. (1995). Brain imaging and language disorders. Paper presented at the Annual Conference of the American Speech-Language-Hearing Association, Orlando, FL.

Hamlet, S.L. (1989). Dynamic aspects of lingual propulsive activity in swallowing. *Dysphagia, 4,* 136–145.

Hamlet, S.L., Stone, M., & Shawker, T. (1988). Posterior tongue grooving in deglutition and speech: Preliminary observations. *Dysphagia, 3* (1), 1–10.

Ishikawa, H., Ishii, Y., Ono, T., Makimoto, K., Yamamoto, K., Torizuka, K. (1983). Evaluation of gray-scale ultrasonography in the investigation of oral and neck mass lesions. *Journal of Oral Maxillofacial Surgery, 41,* 775–781.

Kahrilas, P.J., & Logemann, J.A. (1993). Volume accommodation during swallowing. *Dysphagia, 8,* 259–265.

Kassel, E., Keller, A., & Kuchorczyk, W. (1989). MRI of the floor of the mouth, tongue and orohypopharynx. *Radiologic Clinics of North America, 27* (2), 331–351.

Kelsey, C.A., Hixon, T.J., & Minifie, F.D. (1969). Ultrasonic measurement of lateral pharyngeal wall displacement, *IEEE Transactions on Biomedical Engineering, 16* (2), 1443–1447.

Kenny, D.J., Casas, M.D., & McPherson, K.A. (1989). Correlation of ultrasound imaging of oral swallow with ventilatory alterations in cerebral palsied and normal children. *Dysphagia, 4,* 16–28.

Kenyon, C., Cala, S.J., Watkin, K.L., Macklem, P.T., & Rochester, D.F. (1993). Three-dimensional ultrasonography of a human diaphragm model [Abstract]. *European Respiratory Journal, 6* (Suppl. 17), 1357.

Kim, W., Buchholz, D.W., Kumar, A., Donner, M.W., & Rosenbaum, A.E. (1987). Magnetic resonance imaging for evaluating neurogenic dysphagia. *Dysphagia, 2,* 40–45.

Langmore, S.E., Schatz, K. & Olson, N. (1988). Fiberoptic endoscopic examination of swallowing: A new procedure. *Dysphagia, 2,* 216–219.

Lin, S., Chen, J., Kahrilas, P.J., & Hertz, P. (1994). Three-dimensional animation of the oropharyngeal swallow. *Radiology, 193* (P), 446.

Logemann, J.A. (1983). *Evaluation and treatment of swallowing disorders.* San Diego, CA: College-Hill Press.

Logemann, J.A. (1993). *A manual for videofluoroscopic evaluation of swallowing* (2nd ed.). Austin, TX: Pro-Ed.

Logemann, J.A., Kahrilas, P.J., Begelman, J., Dodds, W.J., & Pauloski, B.R. (1989). Interactive computer program for biomechanical analysis of videoradiographic studies of swallowing. *American Journal of Roentgenology, 153,* 277–280.

Lufkin, R.B., Wortham, D.F., Dietrich, R.B., Hoover, L.A., Larsson, S.G., Kangarloo, H., & Hanafee, W.N. (1986). Tongue and oropharynx findings on MRI. *Radiology, 161,* 69–75.

Miller, J.L. & Watkin, K.L. (1995). Evaluation of US image echodensities during contraction of the lingual musculature. *Canadian Acoustics, 23,* 103–104.

Miller, J.L. & Watkin, K.L. (1996a). Quantitative detection of ultrasound echo intensities: Applications in the evaluation of the lingual musculature during swallowing [Abstract]. *Dysphagia, 11* (2), 167.

Miller, J.L., & Watkin, K.L. (1996b). Color flow doppler ultrasound of lingual hemodynamics: A preliminary study [Abstract]. *Dysphagia, 11* (2), 158.

Muz, I., Mathog, R., Miller, P., Rosen, R., & Borreo, J. (1987). Detection and quantification of laryngotracheopulmonary aspiration with scintigraphy. *Laryngoscope, 97,* 1180–1185.

Ostry, D.J., Flanagan, J.R., Feldman, A.G., & Munhall, K.G. (1991). Human jaw motion control in mastication and speech. In J. Requin & G.E. Stelmach (Eds.), *Tutorials in motor neuroscience.* NATA ASI Series D (Vol. 62, pp. 535–543). Boston: Kluwer Academic Publishers.

Potratz, J.E., Dengel, G., Robbins, J., & Brooks, R. (1993). Movement analysis of oropharyngeal dysphagia: A computer-assisted approach. *Journal of Medical Speech-Language Pathology, 1,* 61–69.

Shawker, T.H. Stone, M., & Sonies, B.C. (1984). Sonography of speech and swallowing. In R.C. Saunders & M.C. Hill (Eds.), *Ultrasound Annual* (pp. 237–260). New York: Raven Press.

Shawker, T., Sonies, B., Hall, T.E., & Baum, B. (1984). Ultrasound analysis of tongue, hyoid and larynx activity during swallowing. *Investigative Radiology, 19* (2), 82–86.

Shawker, T., Sonies, B., Stone, M. & Baum, B. (1983). Real-time ultrasound visualization of tongue movement during swallowing. *Journal of Clinical Ultrasound, 11,* 485–489.

Silver, K.H., & van Nostrand, D. (1991). Scintigraphic detection of salivary aspiration: Description of a new diagnostic technique and case reports. *Dysphagia, 7,* 45–49.

Silver, K.H., & van Nostrand, D. (1994). The use of scintigraphy in the management of patients with pulmonary aspiration. *Dysphagia, 9,* 107–115.

Smith, W.L., Erenberg, A., Nowak, A., & Franken, E.A. (1985). Physiology of sucking in the normal term infant using real-time ultrasound. *Radiology, 156,* 379–381.

Sonies, B.C., Ekman, E.F., Andersson, H.C., Adamson, M.D., Kaler, S.G., Markello, T.C., & Gahl, W.A. (1990). Swallowing dysfunction in nephropathic cystinosis. *New England Journal of Medicine 323,* 565–570.

Sonies, B.C., Parent, L.J., Morrish, K., & Baum, B.J. (1988). Evaluation of swallowing pathophysiology. *Otolaryngologic Clinics of North America, 21,* 638–648.

Sonies, B.C., Stone, M., & Shawker, T. (1984). Speech and swallowing in the elderly. *Journal of Gerontology, 3*, 115–123.

Sonies, B.C., & Wang, C. (1994). Ultrasound doppler spectral analysis of hyoid bone movement during swallow: A preliminary study. Paper presented at the Dysphagia Research Society, McLean, VA.

Sonies, B.C., Wang, C., & Sapper, D. (1996). Assessment of hyoid bone movement during swallowing by use of ultrasound duplex-doppler imaging [Abstract]. *Dysphagia, 11* (2), 162.

Stone, M., & Shawker T.H. (1986). An ultrasound examination of tongue movement during swallowing. *Dysphagia, 1*, 78–83.

Wang, C., & Sonies, B.C. (1995). Methodology for three-dimensional reconstruction of the tongue surface from ultrasound images. Proceedings from the International Society for Optical Engineering, San Diego, CA.

Watkin, K.L., Baer, L.H., Jones, R., Mathur, S., Hakim, S., Diout., I. Nuwayhid, B., & Khalife, S. (1993). Three-dimensional reconstruction of freely acquired two-dimensional medical ultrasonic images. *Volume Image Processing*, 59–62.

Watkin, K.L., Baer, L.H., Mathur, S., Jones, R., Hakim, S., Diout, I., Nuwayhid, B., & Khalife, S. (1993). Three-dimensional reconstruction and enhancement of freely acquired 2D medical ultrasonic images. *IEEE- Canadian Electrical and Computer Engineering*, [proceedings] 1188–1195.

Watkin, K.L., Mathur, S., Baer, L.H., Jones, R., Hakim, S., Diout, I., Nuwayhid, B., & Khalife, S. (1993). Enhancement of 3D and multiple 2D images using a dedicated graphics workstation. *Volume Image Processing*, 153–156.

Watkin, K.L., & Miller, J.L. (1996a). Lateral pharyngeal wall motion during swallowing: Analysis of B/M-mode ultrasound imaging [Abstract]. *Dysphagia, 11* (2), 161.

Watkin, K.L., & Miller, J.L. (1996b). 3D Ultrasonic imaging of the tongue—volume rendering, surface modelling and volume estimation [Abstract]. Submitted to Dysphagia Research Society.

Watkin, K.L. & Myre, R. (1989). Three-dimensional reconstruction of real time ultrasonic scans. *IEEE Ultrasonics Symposium, 1*, 58–59.

Watkin, K.L., Nuwayhid, B., & Khalife, S. (1991). Three-dimensional assessment of a fetal phantom. *Medical Informatics (Europe), 10*, 527–531.

Watkin, K.L., & Rubin, J.M. (1989). Three-dimensional reconstruction of ultrasonic images of the tongue. *Journal of the Acoustical Society of America, 85* (1), 496–499.

Weber, F., Woolridge, M.W., & Baum, J.D. (1986). An ultrasonographic study of the organization of sucking and swallowing by newborn infants. *Developmental Medicine and Child Neurology, 28*, 19–24.

Wein, B., Böckler, R., & Klajman, S. (1991). Temporal reconstruction of sonographic imaging of disturbed tongue movements. *Dysphagia, 6*, 135–139.

Index